# Women, Work, and Health:
# Challenges to Corporate Policy

# WITH CONTRIBUTIONS BY

Edward J. Bernacki, M.D.
  United Technologies Corporation

John D. Blum, J.D.
  Harbridge House

Robert M. Clyne, M.D.
  American Cyanamid Company

Donna Morrison, R.N.; Carmen Moynehan; Stanley P. deLisser; William Wanago, M.D.
  The Executive Health Examiners Group

Jean F. Duff
  General Health Corporation

Joyce C. Hogan, Ph.D.
  Advanced Research Resources Organization

Bruce W. Karrh, M.D.
  E. I. DuPont de Nemours

Ann Lebowitz
  Boston University Health Policy Institute

Richard R. Reilly, Ph.D.
  American Telephone and Telegraph Company

Jeanne M. Stellman, Ph.D.
  Women's Occupational Health Resource Center

Nina G. Stillman, J.D.
  Vedder, Price, Kaufman and Kammholz

Diana Chapman Walsh
  Boston University Center for Industry and Health Care

Leon J. Warshaw, M.D.
  Equitable Life Assurance Society of the United States, on loan to the Office of the Mayor, City of New York

INDUSTRY AND HEALTH CARE 8

# Women, Work, and Health: Challenges to Corporate Policy

EDITED BY
**Diana Chapman Walsh**
**Richard H. Egdahl**

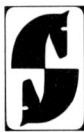
Springer-Verlag   New York

Springer Series on Industry and Health Care
Richard H. Egdahl, M.D., Ph.D.
Diana Chapman Walsh, M.S.
Center for Industry and Health Care
Boston University Health Policy Institute
53 Bay State Road
Boston, Massachusetts 02215

Springer-Verlag New York Inc.
175 Fifth Avenue
New York, NY 10010

**Library of Congress Cataloging in Publication Data**

Main entry under title:

Women, work and health.

   (Industry and health care ; 8)
   Bibliography: p.
   Includes index.
   1. Women—Diseases. 2. Occupational diseases.
3. Women's health services. 4. Women—Employment.
I. Walsh, Diana Chapman. II. Egdahl, Richard
Harrison.
RC963.6.W65W65    658.3′82    80-11369

All rights reserved.

No part of this book may be translated or reproduced in any form without written permission from Springer-Verlag.

The use of general descriptive names, trade names, trademarks, etc. in this publication, even if the former are not especially identified, is not to be taken as a sign that such names, as understood by the Trade Marks and Merchandise Marks Act, may accordingly be used freely by anyone.

© 1980 by Springer-Verlag New York Inc.

Printed in the United States of America.

9 8 7 6 5 4 3 2 1

ISBN 0-387-90478-6 Springer-Verlag New York Heidelberg Berlin
ISBN 3-540-90478-6 Springer-Verlag Berlin Heidelberg New York

# Contents

I. Context and Current Issues

    1. **Genesis and Highlights of a Conference**
       *Diana Chapman Walsh*    3

    2. **Overview: The Health of Working Women**
       *Ann Lebowitz*    27

II. Physical Conditioning, Strength, and Stamina

    3. **The State of the Art of Strength Testing**
       *Joyce C. Hogan*    75

    4. **Moving Women into Outside Craft Jobs**
       *Richard R. Reilly*    99

III. Social Conditioning and the Culture of the Corporation

    5. **Changing Roles and Mental Health in Women**
       *Jean F. Duff*    115

## Contents

6. **Employee Health Services for Women Workers**
   Leon J. Warshaw                                     132

7. **Special Needs of Women in Health Examinations**
   Donna Morrison, Carmen Moynehan, Stanley P.
   deLisser, and William Wanago                        145

8. **Sex Discrimination in Group Pensions**
   John D. Blum                                        156

## IV. Reproductive Potential and Possible Occupational Hazards

9. **A Legal Perspective on Workplace Reproductive Hazards**
   Nina G. Stillman                                    171

10. **The Biology of Toxic Effects on Reproductive Outcomes**
    Jeanne M. Stellman                                 179

11. **Evaluation and Control of Embryofetotoxic Substances**
    Bruce W. Karrh                                     190

12. **Fetotoxicity and Fertile Female Employees**
    Robert M. Clyne                                    198

13. **The Control of Hazardous Exposures in the Workplace**
    Edward J. Bernacki                                 208

## V. Pregnancy and Maternity Leave

14. **A Legal Perspective on Pregnancy Leave and Benefits**
    Nina G. Stillman                                   213

15. **Non-Medical Issues Presented by the Pregnant Worker**
    Leon J. Warshaw                                    231

## VI. Issues for the Future

### 16. Challenges to Corporate Policy
*Diana Chapman Walsh*     245

## Appendix: Conference Participants     257

# CONTEXT AND CURRENT ISSUES

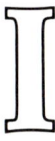

# Genesis and Highlights of a Conference

*Diana Chapman Walsh*

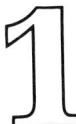

As the principal payer for the health care used by employees and their families, large industrial corporations in the United States have the leverage—and the incentive—to bring about change in the health care delivery system. Previous volumes in the Industry and Health Care series have examined this thesis and the evidence that some companies are at least beginning to test their influence in hopes of containing health care costs. But in relation to the health of women employees, many corporations seem more buffeted by social forces than actively or deliberately leading change. They cannot ignore these forces. They must either set explicit policies or confront individual cases willy-nilly and possibly paint themselves into a policy corner they may later wish to escape.

As women enter the work force in unprecedented and increasing numbers, the health issues surrounding fertility, pregnancy, and childbearing take on increasing salience for employers. These tend to overshadow a set of somewhat more remote but no less real questions concerning the physical and social conditioning of the sexes and how this conditioning interacts with the culture of the corporation to subvert the national goal of equal employment opportunity. Chapter 2 describes the current status in the United States of women, work, and health, and establishes the boundary conditions for this and subsequent chapters.

Fundamentally at issue in the case of pregnancy is a tension between two important social objectives—equality of opportunity on one hand, and, on the other, protection against occupational assaults on reproductive health. In theory, of course, and to some extent in reality, reproductive health is an androgynous issue. Indeed, the male's reproductive system may be more susceptible to chemically induced sterility than is the female's, and the possible transmission of birth defects through the male has yet to be established. Only a woman, however, can "bring a living embryo or fetus into the workplace," where it may be exposed to known or unsuspected fetotoxic substances. Once she is pregnant—even and perhaps especially in the first few weeks, before she can know she is pregnant—the employee's presence can pose medical, legal, and personnel policy problems to challenge the even-handed management of equal employment opportunity.

The pregnancy issues intersect the cultural ones because feminists argue that the line is very fine between benign protection of women and their unborn children and the malign overprotection by men that has "kept women in their place." In contrast, corporate attorneys opt for conservative management policy on fertile women employees who are subject to toxic exposures. They argue that a mother-to-be cannot waive the rights of her unborn child and warn that the company's legal liability could be extensive in the event of an occupationally linked deformity. The medical profession, for its part, prefers to counsel caution in the management of pregnancy generally, the more so in the presence of substances whose prenatal toxic effects are still not fully known.

Into this already complex equation, Congress recently introduced yet another variable—the Pregnancy Disability Act of 1978, Public Law 95–555. The purview and legislative history of this law are outlined in the box and discussed in chapter 15; questions and concerns flowing from it were the immediate stimulus to the conference on which this volume is based. If maternity leave is to be handled like any other disability, then how is *medical disability* to be defined with respect to pregnancy, and by whom? Will the law change the relationships between corporations and local private physicians? What accommodations does the law require of employers whose preexisting maternity leave policies are more flexible or generous than required by the new statute, and is there a danger that their women employees will be the losers as a

## THE PREGNANCY DISABILITY ACT OF 1978

### WHAT

On May 1, 1979, an amendment to Title VII of the Civil Rights Act of 1964 went into effect. Basically, it prohibits employers from discriminating against pregnant workers in any area of employment and benefit programs. Pregnancy and childbirth are to be treated in the same manner as other health problems that interfere with a person's ability to perform his/her assigned task.

### WHY

Since only female workers can become pregnant, discrimination based on pregnancy was seen as discrimination based on sex, specifically prohibited in the civil rights legislation.

### WHERE IS THIS AMENDMENT APPLICABLE

All employers with at least fifteen employees and engaged in interstate commerce must comply.

A company without medical and hospital plans will not be required to begin them.

### IMPLEMENTATION

*Employers cannot:*

- Require a written medical statement of disability for pregnancy unless also required for other disability claims.
- Require a worker to remain on leave until after the birth, even if she has been absent from work because of the pregnancy and then recovers.
- Eliminate a job previously held by a pregnant worker on leave unless she informs the employer she does not intend to return after the birth.
- Refuse to hire a pregnant woman merely because she is pregnant, if she can perform major functions of the job.
- Reduce other benefits to pay added cost of including pregnancy in full benefits package until October 31, 1979, or until expiration of the collective bargaining agreement, whichever is later.
- Require special waiting periods for eligibility for pregnancy benefits if not required for other disabilities.

*Employers can:*

- Refuse benefits if a woman was already pregnant when hired *and* if company also denies medical and hospital coverage for employees with other preexisting conditions.
- Elect not to provide hospital and medical benefits for an abortion not performed to save the woman's life, *but* the employer must provide sick leave or disability benefits for voluntary abortions.

consequence? If so, how will the new policy be implemented? What will be the incremental cost for those firms now required to catch up?

## Genesis of the Conference

With these and other questions arising in anticipation of the effective date of the new pregnancy law, April 1979, the Center for Industry and Health Care of Boston University convened a conference to discuss the law's implications for employers and their women employees, and to place it within the broader context of the special health problems of women workers. The background papers at the core of this volume were commissioned and circulated in advance of the meeting, itself a give-and-take discussion among forty-five invited experts whose names and affiliations appear in the appendix.

To structure the discussion, the sponsors developed an agenda following a crude notion of the life cycle of a working woman, from entry into the work force and career advancement through fertility-related issues, then pregnancy, childbirth, and job reentry. Issues of retirement were touched upon glancingly, with the thought they are sufficiently complex to warrant a separate conference in the future. Throughout, the focus kept sharply on the *health* problems *specific* to women *employees,* despite the strong correlation between health and the social, economic, legal, and cultural environment within which women work. Still, the sharp focus was necessary, not to minimize the impact of socioeconomic issues, but to conserve time and energy for the sufficiently challenging problems related specifically to physical and emotional health.

The agenda began with some questions concerning physical conditioning and preemployment testing for stamina and strength; proceeded to issues of social conditioning and the impact of the corporate environment on the health and mental health of women workers; moved on to the issues surrounding fertility and then pregnancy. The life cycle theme served as a rough organizational framework to aid in unraveling a tangled skein of interrelated issues. Conceptually, it has serious shortcomings, arising from the fact that fertility and childbearing ability are not so much episodes in working women's lives as the essential distinction between the sexes. But the life cycle approach does avoid the "anatomy-is-destiny" fallacy of equating women's health one-to-one with reproductive potential. This seemed too narrow a view.

Originally, we wondered whether there are important health problems peculiar to women workers aside from fertility and maternity issues. Most scientific knowledge about the effects of environmental hazards draws on experiences with experimental animals or men (not women), but the findings published to date have not revealed important differences between the sexes in the nonreproductive physiological responses to toxic environmental exposures.[1] This and growing evidence of the susceptibility of male fertility might seem to argue for a unisex approach to occupational health except in the realm of maternity and possible exposure of embryos or fetuses. But a third factor intrudes—a demographic consideration cogently developed in Jeanne Stellman's writings,[2] and discussed also by Ann Lebowitz in chapter 2 below. This is the fact that women are and have been occupationally segregated, so that the hazards they face are appreciably different from the hazards typically found in male-dominated workplaces. Women as a group have different occupational health needs because, in the aggregate, their exposures and risks are different.

And so are their mental health needs at work. The chapters by Jean Duff and Leon Warshaw in part III consider the impact on emotional health and social well-being of the interpersonal relations in the corporation and the organization of work. The risk factors for job stress—Duff points out in chapter 5—are things like work overload, work stagnation, role conflict, and lack of autonomy or control—all frustrations that attend the economic and occupational inequities many women workers face. This is the essential thread weaving the health of women at work into the economic, social, and cultural fabric of the workplace, and forming the logical backdrop against which the conference is set. What follows for the balance of this chapter are some highlights of the conference, which also is the source of the discussion sections appearing at the end of subsequent chapters. Quotations are used liberally to illustrate the range and intensity of informed opinion among parties to the debate and to enable readers to form their own judgments.

## Conference Highlights

Held on June 11–12, 1979, in Boston, the meeting began with a discussion of the AT&T effort, described in chapter 4, to train women employees for outside craft work. Telephone pole-climbing school is one small part of a much broader program at AT&T, under the 1973 consent decree outlined in the box, to "make sweeping changes in its hiring and promotion practices to advance the cause of women and other minorities within its walls."[3] And while pole climbing per se is probably of fleeting interest to most working women, it does raise other issues that merit wider concern.

> *I could never climb a pole, and I wonder if a lot of this problem isn't just general conditioning differences between boys and girls, not innate physical ability.*
>
> SUSAN C. KARP<br>Citibank

## CATCHING UP: AT&T UNDER THE CONSENT DECREE

Although Title VII of the Civil Rights Act of 1964 specifically prohibits discrimination in employment on the basis of race, color, sex, national origin, and religion, the government had done little before 1970 to define what constituted discrimination in terms of actual employment practices. EEOC's scrutiny of the Bell System, the largest private employer in the country, indicated that although 55 percent of employees were women, the positions they filled were at the low end of the scale in terms of both pay and responsibility. At issue was whether AT&T's compliance with Title VII should be evaluated with reference simply to numbers of women employed or also to their positions in the corporate system. AT&T argued that the firm had made efforts to provide equal opportunity and cited such examples as a special task force established in 1970 to examine the use of women in the Bell System and an "Early Identification" effort to accelerate the upward mobility of female employees who showed potential. The EEOC acknowledged these efforts but held that AT&T should be more aggressive in correcting former inequities rather than simply promising to do better in the future.

On January 18, 1973, AT&T signed a consent decree requiring the company to make major changes in its hiring and promotion of women and minority men. Although not required to admit any past injustices or intentional discrimination, AT&T agreed to pay employees allegedly discriminated against compensatory damages totaling about $18 million, plus an additional $53 million in annual pay increases. Employment percentage goals were then established for each of fifteen job classifications with the intention of hiring more of the sex or race underrepresented in each category. Where women were lacking, a 38 percent work force goal was set with the exception of outside craft jobs where a compromise goal of 19 percent was negotiated.

These goals precipitated problems with the Communications Workers of America Union which represents the bulk of the company's employees. Over the years, AT&T had continually argued over the union's view that seniority should be the principal factor in determining promotion. AT&T had resisted, reserving the right to promote the "best qualified" person based on an evaluation of skills and performance, but had reached a compromise with the union, agreeing to use seniority as a "deciding factor" if two equally qualified employees were being considered for a promotion. Obviously, the government's standards for proportional representation would seriously undermine the accommodation reached between management and labor. To the union's dismay, an "affirmative-action override" was established as a legal solution, allowing AT&T to promote a "basically qualified" person rather than a "best qualified" one, if the interests of the Civil Rights Act were to be served.

> When an evaluation conducted by the Government Coordinating Committee as overseer indicated that AT&T was not moving rapidly enough toward the fulfillment of the consent standard, a supplemental order was signed in 1975 ordering AT&T to speed up their remedial activities, pay compensation, and attempt to interest more women in craft jobs. By the following year, over 90 percent of the goals were met. In January 1979 the decree expired. At that time the government found AT&T in substantial compliance with the law. Negotiations between AT&T and the government are currently under way and expectations are high that a permanent agreement will be reached.
>
> AT&T's experience has implications for many United States businesses. Whatever the reasons for women's traditional predominance in lower level positions, the government has insisted through this consent decree on remedial action and has demonstrated a willingness to oversee its implementation.
>
> Sources: Carol J. Loomis, "AT&T in the Throes of 'Equal Employment,'" Fortune (January 15, 1979). Phyllis Wallace, ed., Equal Employment Opportunity and the AT&T Case, (Cambridge, Mass.: M.I.T. Press, 1976).

*There's no question that conditioning is a big part of this. Working with the Bell System, I've found that a lot of women entering outdoor jobs are doing so because they've been automated out of other work. Many are in grotesque physical condition, mostly because they've been in sedentary jobs. So we set out to develop a program to give them physical training, a better chance of success on the job, less likelihood of an accident, and a better chance at self-improvement and self-acceptance. I believe this kind of activity is going to expand in industry as an affirmative step. But other than AT&T, Exxon, and a few others, it's a step that's not being taken, even though it's essential to safe performance in physically demanding work.*

JOYCE C. HOGAN<br>Advanced Research Resources Organization

## Telephone Poles and Corporate Ladders: Conditioning for the Climb

However remote the pole-climbing case may seem, it provides a metaphor that can be carried close to home. The extra physical conditioning that Joyce Hogan envisages for women pole climbers is an analogue to the mental conditioning that Jean Duff discusses in reference to women's "learned helplessness" and consequent susceptibility to depression. AT&T, under duress, went to considerable lengths and expense to make it easier for women to climb telephone poles—by instituting remedial training, adapting the climbing tool to better suit a woman's physique, and contemplating the modification of the work environment itself by, for example, burying telephone wires underground.

Parallel questions arise concerning how far industry in general is expected to, or should, go to facilitate women's entry into a man's world. What, if any, alterations should be made in the "tools" used in climbing the corporate ladder, in the standards by which proficiency is measured there, and in the environment of the workplace and in the design of jobs to make them more accessible to women? AT&T's consent decree insulated the firm to some extent from effective legal action for reverse discrimination, but that remains as a philosophical and often an emotional issue, if not always a pressing legal one:

> *If we take the attitude that we're going to have specialists for jobs, we're abetting discrimination. It's not the real world to say we'll have a special category of people who climb poles. Let's not dispense with the men's attitudes too quickly. They resent the idea that women do only part of the job or that the job is being modified in some way to make it easier for women.*
>
> ROBERT M. CLYNE
> *American Cyanamid*

> *I have to agree. In this "me-now" world of equal pay for equal work, I've seen problems arise when a person comes back to lighter work after a heart attack or some other disabling disease. Fellow workers are sympathetic for about twenty-four hours, but after that some of them begin to grumble that "people should earn their pay" and "if I'm going to do his work I want some extra money."*
>
> WILLIAM E. R. GREER
> *Gillette*

Joan S. Ward, a British ergonomist,* argues on similar grounds that "sex discrimination is essential in industry":

*Ergonomics is "the study of operations and equipment to take into account human and mental needs."[4] It is a multidisciplinary approach to person-machine relationships combining anthropometry, psychology, physiology, and engineering through which industry hopes to maximize safety, efficiency, and comfort.[5]

> I approve of the concept of "fitting the job to the worker," and if workers are to be of either sex, then jobs must be designed accordingly. But I do not consider that equal opportunity necessarily means that all jobs and their associated equipment must be designed to suit all workers, whether they are men or women. If this course is pursued then equipment would have to be designed with the smallest, weakest woman in mind—and that would certainly discriminate against the tallest, strongest male.[6]

The standard justification for some measure of reverse discrimination is the one the courts have used to uphold the legality of AT&T's affirmative action program: that "it seems 'reasonably calculated' to help undo the effects of past wrongs and move society toward a day in which the distribution of jobs will no longer be affected by discrimination."[7] How far ahead that day lies is a matter for conjecture. Edward J. Bernacki of United Technologies Corporation sees it on the horizon:

> *The earlier people can start on the corporate ladder, the better their chances of getting to the top. Women, because of childbearing and rearing, usually don't get onto the ladder until their late twenties or early thirties. Consequently, they have fewer opportunities to gain the experience needed to assume increasingly important roles within a corporation. If industry can provide services, such as child care centers, to enable women to both work and take care of their parental responsibilities it would increase their chances of getting into more senior positions.*

The corporate tracking system is part of a socialization process that begins long before the first day on the first job. Even if women were to set off in the track at age twenty, some research indicates that they would still start behind in the habits of mind and skills that seem to be essential to a successful career.[8] Other researchers doubt that difficulty in achieving success resides in the woman's personality and point instead to powerful "structural" obstacles, "such as the constraints imposed by roles and the effects of opportunity, power and numbers," in the words of Rosabeth Moss Kanter. Her book, *Men and Women of the Corporation*,[9] attributes the problems facing women managers to "powerlessness, not sex"—behavioral traits that are typical of people placed in the position of "tokens." She also observes that if women are less engaged in or committed to their jobs, there is often less to the jobs in terms of intrinsic interest or opportunity.

This debate echoes one among social scientists in the 1960s as to whether a disabling "culture of poverty" (involving low aspirations, unwillingness to plan for the future, and other passive or self-defeating attitudes or behaviors) is passed from one poor generation to the next,[10] or whether instead the attitudes, planning horizons, and distinctive values of poor people are a positive adaptation to inescapable and extremely harsh life circumstances.[11] The persistence in various forms of the debate over the essential differences among subpopulations (by gender, income, race, age, religion, nationality, and so on) attests to the complexity of the issues involved in affirmative action. Compounding this problem is a shortage of role models:

> *I wish we behavioral scientists had the data base of the pole-climbing trainers who can measure accidents and successful climbing quite adequately. Most women working now have few role models and lack experience with balancing several functions at once—mother, worker, wife. These are not skills that drop out of the sky. It will take several generations to learn them.*
>
> JEAN F. DUFF<br>General Health

To what lengths, then, should industry go to redress the social imbalance for women? Is this a problem that industry can solve and, more particularly, does the corporate ladder pose *health* problems for women that corporate medical departments should be addressing?

> *The problems are not so much medical as social—interpersonal relations on the job and stresses that come from things like arranging adequate child care. Unless we get behavioral scientists involved, we're going to focus on physical organs and miss the essence of these all-too-real problems. For example, with two-career families the crunch comes with the relocation process: whose job is more important? I've seen every possible complex of solutions, including divorce and, in two instances, suicide. So this is a very serious health matter that should be addressed through the employee assistance unit or any available mechanism.*
>
> LEON J. WARSHAW<br>Equitable Life

Employee assistance programs are the focus of another volume in the Industry and Health Care series, which traces their progression from rather narrow initial concerns—alcoholism or substance abuse control, for example—to the much broader goals that many pursue now. Comprehensive programs currently include financial counseling, family counseling, and sometimes child care services:

> *I predict that employee assistance programs are going to take on more and more social responsibility, but this raises a serious question. For companies to take their shareholder responsibilities seriously, there is a real dilemma where their obligation to provide more and more services clashes with the competing need to be rigorous concerning cost-benefit ratios. This is a question for women and men alike, because we do have essentially equal opportunity to buy shares in America's corporations.*
>
> GLEN WEGNER<br>Boise Cascade

In essence, this is the point that Christopher D. Stone and other writers make: that "in the giant, broadly held corporation . . . the 'charitable' gestures . . . all the compromises management makes with profits . . . do not come out of their own pockets," and could in theory therefore result over an extended period of time in "a serious distortion in the pattern of resource use."[12] Stone's position on the corporation's role in society is generally provocative, and he observes dryly that "as a practical matter, the risks of corporate 'largesse' getting so out of hand seem rather small."[13] Milton Friedman, perhaps the strongest exponent of the "proper role of competitive capitalism," would certainly disagree. The question raised by Dr. Wegner is a complicated one.

## Catch–22, Double-Edged Swords, and Other Constraints on Management

In addition to the climbing images related to poles and corporate ladders, we find earth-bound metaphors as well. Catch–22 is a recurrent theme, or Hobson's Choice, which amounts to the same thing—and double-edged swords. On occasion, for example, employers have been held liable for injuries sustained by job applicants in a preemployment test. One employee who failed an examination for a job transfer then went to the state human rights commission and demanded disability benefits on grounds that his failure proved him handicapped.

Whether the new pregnancy disability law will be a double-edged sword for women is hotly contested. There seem to be some adverse trade-offs (requirements for documentation, probationary periods, and the like) for women whose employers already had liberal maternity policies, or who were adequately covered under a collectively bargained plan—still a small minority of working women. But any legal-regulatory attempt to establish homogeneous standards tends to fall indiscriminately on the "good actors" side-by-side with the "bad." It also generally reflects a series of compromises and political accommodations on the way to passage that make the final form less than ideal from everyone's vantage point. So it is with the new pregnancy law:

> *Feminists and union groups have done women a disservice by not truly acquainting them with the trade-offs implied in this law. It's a loss to white-collar women, for example. Prior to the change in the law, many white-collar jobs, such as banking, had a six-month or more unpaid maternity leave, but only fifteen days' paid sick leave and another fifteen days' unpaid leave. Now the law requires the more limited sick leave policy for maternity, as well as more stringent reporting requirements. It may be a rude awakening.*
>
> NINA G. STILLMAN<br>Vedder, Price, Kaufman and Kammholz

> *I disagree. The majority of women who work in banks are tellers. What does an unpaid leave mean to a teller? These jobs are revolving doors. I see this law as a major breakthrough, a step toward not penalizing women for having babies, the beginning of a national policy on childbearing and the employment of women. But it doesn't go far enough. The big companies with existing labor union contracts will have to comply and probably already do; the smaller ones with the part-time and short-term jobs in which most women work offer them no benefits now and will not have to start.*
>
> JEANNE M. STELLMAN<br>Women's Occupational Health Resource Center

There is fairly general agreement, though, that the law's full impact—good and bad—will remain ambiguous during a necessary "shake-down period" of several years' duration. Afterward, there may develop a consensus on the needs for refinement in directions still largely unforeseen.

Another two-edged sword is change in technological processes—automating AT&T's women out of desk jobs and onto telephone poles, creating for medical directors not only a moving target but also an escalating and unpredictable arsenal. Constantly evolving industrial processes bring new substances into the workplace, and thus new problems for medical directors, but they also bring a continually expanding scientific data base and successive refinements in measurement techniques. These changes tend to undermine the very definition of the nature and scope of the problem of protecting women and their unborn children from occupational hazards.

*We're caught by our own advancing technology. We've become more sophisticated and technologically oriented, thus creating some problems; and we've also found that as our analytical capabilities increase, so too does our ability to detect materials. That's the major reason why industry has objected to OSHA's proposed carcinogen standards. The "lowest level feasible" of exposure to a carcinogen could become a moving target never to be reached. Ten years ago we were measuring things in parts per million; now it's parts per billion and parts per trillion.*

BRUCE W. KARRH
*DuPont*

Optimism and pessimism co-mingle in corporate views of the contribution science and technology can make in mitigating the health problems of women workers. There is distress at the limitation on scientific techniques and knowledge:

*We do not know of a single chemical substance that is totally safe. We could test until doomsday and even study populations over periods of years, but at this stage of our technology we still would not know that a material has no adverse effect. We can get closer and closer to that end, but we cannot reach it today. Virtually every material is suspect to some extent.*

ERNEST M. DIXON
*Celanese*

There is concern that occupational health problems are seriously exacerbated by more general issues of environmental quality:

*We are dealing with multiple chemicals with synergistic effects—chemicals not only in the workplace, but in the diet, the home, and the outside environment. The problems in industry are relatively focused but still tremendously complex.*

LEON J. WARSHAW

And there is frustration at the difficulty of setting research priorities:

*Six or eight years ago, would any one have said that we should be suspicious of vinyl chloride? I think not. We know there is a dose-effect relationship in almost everything in the environment. Enough water will kill you. Enough of a carcinogen, even a weak one, will eventually kill you. But you might have to live to be 185 years old before you develop the cancer. We see lists from*

*NIOSH\* and we develop our own lists, but we would have to have the wisdom of Solomon multiplied a thousandfold.*

ROBERT M. CLYNE

On the other hand, there is some satisfaction at the progress being made toward rational, systematic control of potential problems:

*Let's not overstate our ignorance. There's a whole lot we do know about many potentially hazardous occupational agents. Sound industrial hygiene and medical surveillance programs can be initiated to assure workers of their safety when they work with these substances.*

EDWARD J. BERNACKI

And there is a feeling that one ought not to lose a sense of balance:

*We should keep things in perspective. NIOSH has recently published a list of agents with reproductive effects, fifty-nine different materials beginning with A for aldrin and ending with Z for zinc oxide, and also a two-inch-thick booklet of teratogens.\*\* Yet Dr. Karrh tells us that DuPont uses only six of these chemicals, five of which they can control environmentally to below the threshold limit value. American Cyanamid is smaller than DuPont. We use 20,000 chemicals to produce 2,000 products, but only five of the chemicals are in the NIOSH booklet. So we're not talking about hundreds and hundreds of toxic chemicals. We want incontravertible evidence before we act, and we're trying to develop that. It takes time and costs money.*

ROBERT M. CLYNE

## Discrete Professional Perspectives

Perspective can be an important factor in discussions of women's roles. The special health problems of women workers evoke the distinct and sometimes conflicting world views of different professions: the biochemical researcher, the corporate attorney, the occupational physician, the community physician, and, of course, the woman worker herself. An MIT biochemistry professor characterizes the problems at the molecular level as "at least as confusing" as they are at the levels of regulation and commerce. While he rejects the suggestion that the

---

\*The National Institute of Occupational Safety and Health.
\*\*Fetotoxins responsible for structural deformities.

situation is "hopeless," Christopher Walsh draws a bleak picture of the time and expense involved in tentatively certifying one chemical safe:

> From a scientific point of view, we face probably the most complex set of investigations one could imagine and they are geometrically more so every year. To talk about standards is distracting in the extreme because these are ad hominem standards, whether forty micrograms, ten micrograms, or one part per trillion. No matter what you tell employees, I see no guarantee that ten years from now these will be considered safe standards. There are serious questions about whether any level is safe—to bring up the Delaney problem.* Are dose-responses linear? What are the threshold effects? What is the cumulative build-up? We talk about women of childbearing age in the workplace and tend to say, "Until she is pregnant, it is not a problem," but we don't know what the persistence of residue levels is. Or what the interaction of one chemical or one particulate is with another and what the dwell time will be so that a fetus conceived two years later isn't still at risk. There are fluctuating responses in terms of the susceptibility to toxins of different embryos and fetuses. Most drug-metabolizing enzymes don't show up until the first six months of life, and the capacity for warding off harmful drugs may not be fully established until four years of age.

Independent of these "Byzantine scientific questions" are practical limitations on the nation's laboratory testing capacity, which is growing in anticipation of increased demands, as yet to be stimulated, from the Toxic Substance Control Act of 1976. There are now an estimated 50,000 to 70,000 chemicals used in commercial production; only a fraction have ever been tested for carcinogenicity or mutagenicity. Another 1,000 new chemicals are introduced into commerce each year. The total current capacity to test for carcinogenicity is about 150 to 200 chemicals a year, at a cost per chemical of around $250,000.[15] One government estimate places the cost of the testing to catch up with untested organic chemicals at $12 billion and the annual cost to stay current at $300 million.[16]

---

*The Delaney Amendment to the Food and Drug Act,[14] introduced by Congressman Delaney in 1958, stipulates that "no [food] additive shall be deemed to be safe if it is found . . . after tests which are appropriate for the evaluation of the safety of food additives, to induce cancer in animal or man." Subsequent regulations extended the principle to feed for promoting animal growth and to food colorings. The assumptions behind the clause and the sources of controversy are that the only tolerable exposure level to a carcinogen is zero and that animal tests are sufficient to "establish" carcinogenicity.

**18** Context and Current Issues

> We're going to be in the twenty-second century before we've made much headway. So one makes choices based on bulk production, structures, and exposures expected. But suppose those choices turn out in hindsight not to have been very good and you haven't tested your worst carcinogen until twenty-five years hence. Someone who would like to do toxicological studies faces a major problem in just sorting out the scientific choices.
>
> CHRISTOPHER WALSH

Without benefit of extensive case law, the corporate attorney understands the jury process well enough to sense that management does have legitimate cause for concern.

> It has been asserted that because spontaneous abortions and fetal malformations are common, the level of information needed to prove job-relatedness is high. In theory, I would have to agree. But as a practical matter, these cases are generally tried before juries. If a plaintiff brings a deformed child into the courtroom, a big-name corporate defendant is up against amazing odds, even if it doesn't have the burden of proof. The jurors will assume that the firm can easily afford to pay or can pass on the cost to an insurer. The appellate courts tend to be more realistic, but I can imagine initial awards in the $10.5 million range. Look at the Silkwood case.
>
> NINA G. STILLMAN

The Silkwood case was the first to be tried on the question of the nuclear industry's liability for off-site contamination. In November 1974 Karen Silkwood, a plutonium worker in a plant owned by Kerr-McGee Nuclear Corporation, died in an automobile accident while on her way to a meeting with a reporter from the *New York Times* and a representative of the Oil, Chemical and Atomic Workers Union, allegedly to turn over documents proving that conditions at the plant were unsafe. The documents were never found, but Ms. Silkwood and her apartment had been contaminated by plutonium earlier that month, and her surviving family brought suit against Kerr-McGee, claiming negligence on the company's part for the contamination. The judge in the case accepted the argument by attorneys for the Silkwood family that the nuclear industry is absolutely liable for the escape of low-level radiation and that negligence does not have to be shown. On May 19, 1979, the federal court jury awarded $10.5 million in damages to the Silkwood family. Kerr-McGee announced plans to appeal the verdict.

For an attorney who represents management, Nina Stillman believes, there were—beyond the magnitude of the award—ominous portents in the Silkwood decision:

> In essence, the court found that compliance with existing standards as set forth in government regulations will not insulate employers if the standard turns out to have been inadequate. The Silkwood judge has opted for strict liability, and if that is to become a rule of law, then I would have to advise any chemical manufacturer to take the most conservative approach, which is to ban fertile women entirely. If employers are going to have to pick up a tremendous tab based on hindsight, then they have got to protect themselves in advance to the best of their ability.

Within the doubly ambiguous context of scientific and legal uncertainty, occupational physicians have a dual obligation to their patients and their employers:

> Serious doubts remain about whether the new lead standards will adequately protect a fetus. What are we corporate physicians going to advise women employees? I am sure we will tell them our opinions and what we know of the facts. Perhaps we will offer some advice as to whether we think they should take the risk. And what are we going to advise the employer concerning the legal risks he may be taking?
>
> MARCUS BOND<br>AT&T

Industrial physicians straddle two medical arenas with potential legal liabilities nipping at both heels. On one side is the employer's liability for occupationally related injuries, on the other the potential for medical malpractice suits:

> We're dealing essentially with case law, which is constantly developing and in flux, and that makes it difficult to assess future liability. But one development that gives me pause comes out of two recent New York malpractice cases. The courts held that suits could be entertained against physicians for failing to warn pregnant women adequately about the danger of an abnormal child, in one case because of congenital kidney disease, in the other, Down's syndrome. In each instance, the physician was found negligent in not doing amniocentesis to detect the abnormality so that the woman could have an abortion and avoid the liability and care of a damaged child. Those cases are still in court on appeal, but could be ominous for occupational physicians even

*though they originated elsewhere. What are our legal responsibilities to inform the pregnant or would-be pregnant worker of risks in the workplace? What should we do to monitor a pregnancy for abnormality and what steps can we take to anticipate problems and spare the burden on the woman and the family of having a deformed child? These are open-ended questions.*

LEON J. WARSHAW

Perhaps because of their dual obligations, and a legacy of strained relations with organized labor,[17] occupational physicians seldom seem content to let it go without saying that human and health considerations—and the practice of high-quality medicine—weigh at least as heavily with them as do the economic and legal issues they must face with their employers:

*Our goal is to practice good medicine for everybody who comes into the workplace. A fetus brought into the workplace is just as much our responsibility as is a male or female worker. I would be disturbed to think that anyone might go away believing that this is purely a matter of avoiding economic or legal consequences. As physicians in industry, we're very much concerned with human health matters.*

ROBERT M. CLYNE

*One of the biggest problems is that a certain number of pregnancies are going to involve spontaneous abnormalities. But if a female of childbearing capability has been exposed at work to a known teratogenic compound and subsequently develops an abnormal child, then even if it were one of these "spontaneous" problems that occurs in 5–10 percent of cases, the burden of proof would have shifted to the employer. To prove that occupational exposure was not the cause is all but impossible to do. I would add that the multimillion-dollar lawsuit is not the sole consideration, although I'm sure it has some bearing on the decisions of many companies, including my own. Any abnormal infant produces emotional and financial stress. The thought that you could have prevented this and didn't, or didn't take a prudent enough course, is difficult for a physician to take.*

BRUCE W. KARRH

However actively the corporate medical department may become involved in framing policy to govern pregnancy in the workplace, general community physicians—whether obstetricians or other practitioners—will retain their established roles in the management of their patients' pregnancies. They will therefore need to advise women patients concerning potential risks during the pregnancy and will now also become involved with employers in the certification of disability under the new pregnancy law. The impact of work on perinatal welfare becomes increasingly important with the growth of work-force participation by women. Whether physicians as a group are adequately prepared for their expanding role is a matter of some concern.

> Most women do not work for large corporations with extensive in-house medical departments, nor are they employed in industrial plants with plant physicians and union counselors who can give them guidance and help. So by and large, the task falls to the private physician to assess the situation, look at the problems with understanding, and offer whatever advice our meager scientific knowledge permits. This is the reason ACOG* has developed guidelines, and I commend them to everyone as a first step in addressing a knotty problem.
>
> LEON J. WARSHAW

The ACOG guidelines are described in chapters 2 and 6 and are referenced in the annotated bibliography. Dr. Warshaw chaired the project, which was funded by NIOSH; Dr. Louise Tyrer was another of the seven physicians comprising the project's core panel.

> After practicing obstetrics for over twenty-five years, I'm certainly aware that there exist some concerns and confusion on the part of physicians in regard to signing for a woman's disability. On one hand is the patient who wishes to claim disability and asks the doctor to sign for it although the reasons may or may not be compelling. Yet there are valid concerns about women working late in pregnancy, or concerns that if the woman were to develop a complication and the physician had refused to sign for the disability, there could be a law suit. Very often, therefore, the physician does indeed sign such a statement. On the other hand, the next patient may come in and say, "I wish to continue to work, and they're discriminating against me in saying I should not work; would you please sign a statement validating my capability to work?" The two patients may be very similar but the doctor very often will be inclined to sign both the statements. The ACOG

---

*The American College of Obstetricians and Gynecologists.

> guidelines were developed for this reason; the most important thing is to educate the physician to be totally objective in exercising clinical judgment.
>
> LOUISE B. TYRER
> Planned Parenthood Federation of America

Practicing obstetricians have no incentive to override or second-guess a pregnant patient's feelings concerning her ability to continue work. All the incentives push them to accede to her wishes. Before the enactment of the Pregnancy Disability law, employers had little financial stake in this judgment and in most cases were probably just as glad to have the pregnant woman stop working early lest there be a complication. The employer's stakes increase when the physician's judgment that a woman is disabled effectively commits the employer's funds. Yet it is likely true that few practicing obstetricians have closely followed the implications of the new law.

> When a pregnant patient comes in and says, "Doctor, I don't think I should work any more," with the disability form already filled out, the easiest thing for the obstetrician to do is sign it. You may be hesitant to offend the patient, afraid of losing referrals, or of having unhappy patients. There's also, as much as we may hate to admit it, the fact that medicine is very often an inexact science. We can't be sure the symptomatology of a pregnant patient who works on the assembly line will not be a potential problem. And we certainly would hate to be in a positon where we opted to be less conservative only to have something bad happen later on. So we all tend to be overly cautious, in particular when dealing with pregnant women, because we're then really dealing with two patients. Also, there's the problem that while we may ask a few questions about employment and the kinds of tasks involved on the job, I'm not at all sure most practicing physicians go into enough depth as to the possible hazards of the workplace—especially toxins and physical stresses—to make an informed assessment. Those are just a few of the issues in certifying disability for pregnancy.
>
> KENNETH EDELIN
> University Hospital, Boston

Even if confronted with dramatic inconsistencies, the obstetrician has little reason to assume the role of policeman. Physicians take their patients one at a time and are not generally comfortable with the notion that they should allocate society's scarce resources, whether CAT scans, coronary artery bypass surgery, kidney transplants, or paid disability days. Without limits set by social policy, there is no reason to expect individual physicians or patients to mute their demands for the most that money can buy. It is to a failure of public policy and not to malfeasance or venality that the faulty incentives can be traced.

The role of practicing physicians in pregnancy disability certification is discussed at greater length in chapter 14, where additional quotations from the conference reveal a tension between alarm on the part of some corporate managers that the new pregnancy law will be an invitation to abuse by women workers in collusion with their loyal obstetricians, and equally strong sentiment among women workers that the law will not be abused, or will be no more so than is any insurance program. Time has not yet resolved the debate.

Underlying the debate are divergent assumptions about the woman's own perspective—not only the inflammatory issue of "abuse," but much more fundamental questions concerning her ability to make appropriate choices, reach optimal decisions, and establish priorities when information is severely limited, and her right to do so even if it may mean making a wrong decision. Some physicians express considerable confidence in the judgment of women patients and respect for pregnancy as a constructive motivating force. Others seem to have less, and even some women have doubts.

> The premise behind letting the woman decide is that prospective parents are responsible. My experience from both the legal field and from involvement with Planned Parenthood has shown that, unfortunately, this is not always the case. Knowing of a potential risk, humans will still go ahead and take it: "It's my child, and I'll make the decision . . . I'll take the chance." I'm not sure that's responsible parenthood. People frequently have children without necessarily considering potential hazards such as cigarettes, alcohol, and drugs, yet the hazards inherent in these items have been shown.
>
> NINA G. STILLMAN

And the argument is advanced that the potential legal liability renders the question moot—that the corporation lacks the discretion to permit women to make these judgments for themselves:

> Allowing the decision to be made by the woman is basically at odds with OSHA's premise that you protect employees in spite of themselves. That is clearly seen where employees don't want certain protective measures and the employer is required to force it on them. Longshoremen were violently opposed to wearing

> hard hats, their employers couldn't get them to wear them, and they had wildcat strikes over the issue. However, the court told the employer, in essence, "That's tough. You'll have to bear a wildcat strike, if necessary, in order to protect the workers."
>
> NINA G. STILLMAN

Jeanne M. Stellman, a physical chemist who now heads the Women's Occupational Health Resource Center in New York, finds these arguments unconvincing and suggests, in rebuttal, that a "fetus fetish" or a "myth of perpetual pregnancy" is perhaps being used by a male-controlled culture to see that it remains so. If not, she asks, then how does one account for the tendency to find that when expedient, as during World War II or now in occupations such as nursing where women play essential roles, there is not the same sense of urgency about protecting them and their unborn children:

> We shouldn't establish generic policy on reproductive hazards for women in the ball court of the chemical industry. Let's move over to the health industry and ban women from working with ionizing radiation or dental technicians from working with mercury. Let's remove women from places where they could be exposed to infectious agents that may cause birth defects. In industries where women are essential, suddenly we are not talking about excluding them. Only in heavy industry, where women have begun making some minor inroads toward equal opportunity, does one encounter this very acute consciousness about fetuses. I would like to destroy what I call "the perpetual pregnancy myth," the assumption that anyone fertile and female will inevitably become pregnant.
>
> JEANNE M. STELLMAN

Stellman points out that some 90 percent of the women in the United States are finished with childbearing before the age of 29 and 95 percent by the age of 34, that over 60 percent of married women's pregnancies are planned, and the major source of unplanned pregnancy now is unwed teenagers:

> The vast majority of women at risk for pregnancy don't develop the condition when they're out working—especially the ones who've had to work the second shift, catch two hours' sleep, and get up to send their kids off to school. Most women who've been told of a potential risk to pregnancy from specific occupational exposures will want to cooperate with management in avoiding it. Women don't want to have deformed fetuses. The vast majority

within our society are mature enough to make the appropriate decisions. After all, the child will be theirs, not the company's. Women in heavy industry should be informed of potential risks and given the same freedom of choice accorded men working in similar circumstances.

**Moderator:** *But if you grant that no one can waive the rights of the fetus should an unsuspected chemical turn out to be a problem, then suppose you were retained by American Cyanamid or DuPont to help them come up with a sensible, practical, socially progressive policy—but still a survival policy—what do you suggest they do?*

**Stellman:** *I don't know. I think it's not a good time to be a chemical company.*

The response may be part tongue-in- cheek, but does imply an appreciation of the dilemmas facing chemical manufacturers, if little in the way of concrete help. Jeanne Stellman, of course, knows this; her center does provide concrete help as a clearinghouse of information and technical assistance on women's occupational health problems for working women, management, professionals, and government policymakers.

Others, too, are working at solutions of various sorts—some described or alluded to in subsequent chapters or accessible through an annotated bibliography, available upon request.* The volume is not an exhaustive treatise, but rather, we hope, a timely, balanced, and provocative look at some thorny social and health issues challenging American industry.

Considerably more detail on evolving industrial and public policy affecting occupational health, and many additional references, appear in the first and fourth volumes of the Industry and Health Care series. Chapters 2 through fifteen of the present volume consist of the edited background papers, organized according to the format of the conference. Chapter 2 is a factual repository that lays essential groundwork for the remaining, more specifically focused chapters. Although no papers were read nor narrowly discussed at the meeting, selected excerpts from the transcript have been appended to some of the chapters during the editing process. These appear under the rubric of "discussion" and are included to indicate the diversity of opinion on some of the material in the papers. The "boxes" on various pages are designed to provide a simple, concise overview of specific baseline information. They too are editorial adjuncts, for which the chapter au-

*Center for Industry and Health Care, Boston University, 53 Bay State Road, Boston, MA, 02115.

thors should not be held accountable. Chapter sixteen, finally, attempts to summarize the major issues raised and speculates on some directions future policy may take.

## NOTES

1. Bruce N. Ames, "Identifying Environmental Chemicals Causing Mutations and Cancer," *Science* 204 (May 11, 1979): 587.
2. Jeanne Mager Stellman, *Women's Work, Women's Health* (New York: Pantheon, 1977).
3. Carol J. Loomis, "AT&T in the Throes of 'Equal Employment,' " *Fortune* (January 15, 1979): 45.
4. Nicholas Ashford, *Crisis in the Workplace* (Cambridge, Mass.: MIT Press, 1976): 509.
5. Carl Zenz (ed.), *Occupational Medicine: Principles and Practical Applications* (Chicago: Yearbook Medical Publications, 1975): 423–442.
6. Joan S. Ward, "Sex Discrimination Is Essential in Industry," in *Health of Women at Work: Proceedings of a Symposium Organized by the Society of Occupational Medicine Research Panel* (London: The Royal Society of Medicine, 1976): 1.
7. Loomis, "AT&T," pp. 54–56.
8. Margaret Hennig and Anne Jardin, *The Managerial Woman* (New York: Pocket Books, 1976).
9. Rosabeth Moss Kanter, *Men and Women of the Corporation* (New York: Basic Books, 1977).
10. See, e.g., Daniel P. Moynihan, *The Negro Family* (Washington, D.C.: Office of Policy, Planning and Research, Department of Labor, 1965).
11. See, e.g., Lee Rainwater, "Crucible of Identity," in *The American Negro*, ed. Talcott Parsons and Kenneth Clark (Boston: Houghton Mifflin, 1966).
12. Christopher D. Stone, *Where the Law Ends* (New York: Harper & Row, 1975): 232–233.
13. Ibid., p. 233n.
14. U.S. Code of Federal Regulations 409 (c) (3) (A) and 512 (d) (1) (H).
15. Ames, "Environmental Chemicals," p. 588.
16. Douglas Martin, "Search for Toxic Chemicals in Environment Gets a Slow Start, Is Proving Difficult and Expensive," *Wall Street Journal* (May 9, 1978): 48.
17. See, e.g., Sheldon W. Samuels, "The Problems of Industry-Sponsored Health Programs," in *Background Papers on Industry's Changing Role in Health Care Delivery*, ed. Richard H. Egdahl and Diana Chapman Walsh (New York: Springer-Verlag, 1977): 152–158.

# Overview: The Health of Working Women

Ann Lebowitz

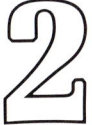

For the first time in history, most American women are employed or actively looking for work. The upsurge of employed women has been both rapid and massive: in less than thirty years, the proportion of women who are employed has risen from one-third to over one-half, far exceeding official Labor Department predictions. As of 1976, women accounted for 38 percent of employees in private industry and 42 percent of the work force as a whole. The long-term ramifications of this for the labor market and for women themselves, collectively and individually, are only beginning to be explored.

Any social phenomenon of these proportions is likely to have multiple causes. Among those that have been invoked are feminism, the falling birth rate, the increase in female-headed households, the explosion of service jobs, federal antidiscrimination legislation, the rise in women's level of education, the effect of inflation on family budgets, and individual recognition of the hazards of relying entirely on a husband's income. We need not try to account fully for what economist Eli Ginzburg, chairman of the National Commission for Manpower Policy, has called "the single most outstanding phenomenon of the century." It is sufficient for our purposes to point out that, whatever other factors are at work, fully two-thirds of employed women in 1976 were unmarried, widowed, divorced, separated, or married to men who earned less than $10,00. In other words, most need their own incomes for simple economic survival.

It may be noteworthy, too, that the typical working woman is statistically likely to have seen her mother enter or reenter the work force at some point during her own childhood. During the postwar period, married women past the prime childbearing years accounted for the greatest increase in female employment; today the greatest increase is occurring among their 25–35-year-old daughters, of whom nearly three-quarters are mothers of dependent children.

Let us look at the conditions of working women's lives, the circumstances they encounter in the labor market, and their consequent labor-market behavior.

## Working Women and the Female Labor Market

### Portrait of American Working Women

The overriding fact of life for most working women is their extensive unpaid household and parental responsibilities. Over half of all mothers with dependent children were in the labor force in March 1978, accounting for approximately two out of every five women workers. Including all those young women who will eventually work while their children are young, and those older women who have previously done so, accounts for the overwhelming majority of American women. Sixty percent of those with children aged 6–17 and nearly 40 percent of those with children below age 3 were working or looking for work in 1978.

Most employed mothers of all ages are married and living with their husbands. A fast-growing minority, however—currently about 20 percent—are divorced, separated, widowed, or never-married. Divorced and separated women are the most likely of all women, including single women, to be in the labor force; nearly two-thirds are employed. Nevertheless, female-headed households are overwhelmingly poor. Such families are 83 percent more likely than male-headed families to pay over one-quarter of their income for rent, considered a particularly telling indicator of economic disadvantage.

*Responsibility for Children*

Who cares for the children of working women? Overwhelmingly, the mothers themselves do. Only about one-quarter of such children aged 3–13 are cared for by adults (except grade school teachers) other than their parents, and when the father participates in child care his contribution is typically less than an hour a day.

Some women strike a compromise between their family responsibilities and their jobs by working while the children are in school; a sizeable number work night shifts, or evenings and weekends, while the father cares for the children.

Women whose children are cared for by others typically make private arrangements, more often than not with a relative; only a minuscule number of children attend day care centers. Working women's child care arrangements, whether or not they involve other adults, are typically makeshift and subject to the child's good health, and they tend to prove less workable during school holidays and vacations.

*Household Responsibilities*

The classic large-scale study of American women's child care and household responsibilities was conducted at Cornell University in the late 1960s, drawing on the responses of 1,300 married women from a wide spectrum of income classes.[1] The investigators found that employed women spend only slightly less time on their home responsibilities than do at-home women. Depending on the number and ages of the children, employed wives' average workweeks vary from 66 to 75 hours. Husbands' contributions vary *only* with the number of hours they devote to their jobs; husbands contribute about 11 hours a week to household work whether or not their wives work and irrespective of the number and ages of children. Women employed full time typically work the equivalent of two full workdays a week more than their husbands. In sum, most working women hold two jobs, one paid and one unpaid.

This pattern is remarkably uniform throughout the female work force. Even women who earn far more than the average female salary tend to have home responsibilities not very different from the average. One can only conjecture about overwork and lack of leisure as contributory factors to emotional and chronic physical illnesses.

*Earnings*

The average married woman who works full-time year-round earns about $8,600, or about 38 percent of the average total family income of $22,631. To put it another way, her husband earns 63 percent more than she does for the same number of hours. (Such a family's standard tax liability, assuming four exemptions, rises about $2,000 as a result of the wife's extra income; if her expenses rise as well, as is likely, she is typically working for a very small—though often crucial—income.) But most two-earner families do not fit this pattern, since the majority of married women work intermittently and/or part-time. The median income of all employed wives is $5,100, closer to 25 percent of average total family earnings.

In general, the lower the family's total income, the higher the proportion earned by the woman. If total family income is under $10,000, the major support of the family tends to be the wife.

## The Female Labor Market and Women's Employment Patterns

When women enter the labor market, what skills, expectations, and restraints do they bring with them, and what opportunities and constraints do they encounter? Though it is impossible to sort out what is cause and what is effect, the situation itself is unmistakable: the labor market is highly segregated by sex.

### Women's Jobs

Despite well-publicized inroads into a number of untraditional occupations, women are still overwhelmingly concentrated in a few occupations regarded as "women's work." Ten occupations account for fully 40 percent of the entire female work force: secretary, retail salesclerk, bookkeeper, private household worker, elementary school teacher, waitress, typist, cashier, sewer and stitcher, and registered nurse. Fully one-third of employed women are clerical workers. By contrast, the ten largest occupations for men employ less than 20 percent of all men.

Segregation by sex is *increasing*, whether viewed over the short term or the long. The record influx of women into the labor force is not serving to reduce occupational segregation because the greatest increases are occurring in precisely those occupations women have been filling all along. The proportion of women who are employed in the leading occupations for women has risen since 1960, and a number of studies have concluded that segregation by sex is as great if not greater now than at the turn of the century. Some analysts conclude, in fact, that the main reason for the huge influx of married women into the labor market is soaring demand in the traditional female occupations. Approximately half the record increase in female employment in 1978 was in clerical and service occupations. Table 1 lists occupations in which women held at least 50 percent of all jobs in 1970; it is striking how many of the occupations listed are almost exclusively female.

**Table 1**
**Occupations in Which Women Hold at Least 50 Percent of Total Jobs, 1970**

| Occupation | Number of Females Employed | Female Employment as Percent of Total Employment in Occupation | Female Employment in Occupation as Percent of Total Female Employment |
|---|---|---|---|
| Home Management Advisors | 5,177 | 95.994 | 0.018 |
| Librarians | 99,851 | 81.944 | 0.345 |
| Dieticians | 36,909 | 91.971 | 0.127 |
| Registered Nurses | 47,563 | 63.829 | 0.164 |
| Clinical Laboratory Technol. & Techn. | 84,641 | 71.960 | 0.292 |
| Dental Hygienists | 14,863 | 94.039 | 0.051 |
| Health Record Technol. & Techn. | 10,283 | 92.108 | 0.035 |
| Therapy Assistants | 2,118 | 65.960 | 0.007 |
| Health Technologists & Technicians | 33,525 | 56.040 | 0.115 |
| Religious Workers | 19,125 | 55.674 | 0.068 |
| Social Workers | 135,813 | 62.695 | 0.469 |
| Teachers, Elementary & Secondary | 1,674,376 | 70.103 | 5.781 |
| Teachers, Prekindergarten & Kindergarten | 122,354 | 97.890 | 0.422 |
| Teachers | 106,393 | 70.290 | 0.367 |
| Dancers | 4,878 | 82.412 | 0.016 |
| Demonstrators | 34,462 | 91.039 | 0.119 |
| Hucksters and Peddlers | 93,064 | 79.161 | 0.321 |
| Bank Tellers | 214,879 | 86.212 | 0.759 |
| Billing Clerks | 87,202 | 82.265 | 0.301 |
| Bookkeepers | 1,255,111 | 81.938 | 4.436 |
| Cashiers | 689,461 | 83.722 | 2.436 |
| Clerical Assistants, Social Welfare | 937 | 78.213 | 0.003 |
| Counter Clerks | 151,605 | 66.630 | 0.535 |
| Enumerators & Interviewers | 50,091 | 77.578 | 0.174 |

(continued)

**Table 1 (Continued)**
**Occupations in Which Women Hold at Least 50 Percent of Total Jobs, 1970**

| Occupation | Number of Females Employed | Female Employment as Percent of Total Employment in Occupation | Female Employment in Occupation as Percent of Total Female Employment |
|---|---|---|---|
| File Clerks | 292,252 | 81.941 | 1.032 |
| Bookkeeping & Billing Machine Operators | 56,565 | 89.405 | 0.195 |
| Calculating Machine Operators | 31,843 | 91.251 | 0.110 |
| Duplicating Machine Operators | 11,526 | 56.876 | 0.039 |
| Key Punch Operators | 244,674 | 89.765 | 0.845 |
| Office Machine Operators | 24,553 | 67.827 | 0.845 |
| Payroll & Timekeeping Clerks | 107,264 | 68.844 | 0.379 |
| Proofreaders | 21,030 | 74.842 | 0.072 |
| Receptionists | 287,053 | 94.764 | 1.014 |
| Secretaries | 2,638,033 | 97.629 | 9.324 |
| Statistical Clerks | 160,269 | 64.281 | 0.553 |
| Stenographers | 119,875 | 93.150 | 0.414 |
| Teacher's Aides | 117,359 | 90.272 | 0.404 |
| Typists | 920,612 | 94.185 | 3.182 |
| Miscellaneous Clerical Workers | 302,267 | 63.656 | 1.044 |
| Not Specified Clerical Workers | 607,437 | 75.248 | 2.099 |
| Clerical & Kindred Workers Allocated | 550,108 | 72.648 | 1.901 |
| Bookbinders | 19,441 | 57.122 | 0.067 |
| Decorators & Window Dressers | 40,251 | 57.534 | 0.139 |
| Clothing Ironers & Pressers | 139,394 | 75.272 | 0.481 |
| Graders & Sorters, Manufacturing | 24,352 | 64.070 | 0.084 |
| Produce Graders & Packers (exc. Farm) | 19,356 | 72.958 | 0.066 |
| Laundry & Drycleaning Operatives | 108,022 | 63.776 | 0.381 |
| Meat Wrappers, Retail Trade | 41,112 | 93.253 | 0.142 |
| Milliners | 1,855 | 90.136 | 0.006 |

| | | | |
|---|---|---|---|
| Packers & Wrappers (exc. Meat & Prod.) | 314,067 | 60.922 | 1.110 |
| Sewers & Stitchers | 812,716 | 93.695 | 2.872 |
| Shoe-making Machine Operatives | 36,419 | 60.213 | 0.125 |
| Solderers | 23,851 | 81.615 | 0.113 |
| Knitters, Loopers, & Toppers | 18,089 | 63.680 | 0.062 |
| Spinners, Twisters, & Winders | 99,222 | 63.612 | 0.342 |
| Weavers | 26,680 | 53.209 | 0.092 |
| Winding Operatives | 30,939 | 50.937 | 0.106 |
| Chambermaids & Maids | 186,660 | 94.863 | 0.645 |
| Cleaners & Charwomen | 252,423 | 57.491 | 0.872 |
| Cooks (exc. Private Household) | 523,485 | 63.148 | 1.809 |
| Food Counter & Fountain Workers | 115,563 | 76.339 | 0.399 |
| Food Service Workers | 246,465 | 75.946 | 0.851 |
| Dental Assistants | 86,309 | 97.883 | 0.298 |
| Health Aides (exc. Nurses) | 100,602 | 84.605 | 0.347 |
| Health Trainees | 16,549 | 93.735 | 0.057 |
| Lay Midwives | 537 | 79.555 | 0.001 |
| Nurse's Aides, Orderlies, & Attendants | 609,022 | 84.825 | 2.105 |
| Practical Nurses | 228,648 | 96.421 | 0.790 |
| Airline Stewardesses | 31,290 | 95.822 | 0.108 |
| Attendants, Personal Service | 37,262 | 62.319 | 0.128 |
| Boarding & Lodging Housekeepers | 5,484 | 71.686 | 0.018 |
| Child-care Workers (exc. Private Household) | 122,062 | 93.013 | 0.421 |
| Hairdressers & Cosmetologists | 424,873 | 90.104 | 1.486 |
| Housekeepers (exc. Private Household) | 74,265 | 71.861 | 0.256 |
| School Monitors | 23,468 | 90.237 | 0.081 |
| Welfare Service Aides | 11,712 | 76.529 | 0.040 |
| Crossing & Bridge Tenders | 23,919 | 57.431 | 0.082 |
| Service Workers (exc. Private Household) | 416,142 | 58.999 | 1.470 |
| Private Household Workers | 1,109,854 | 96.855 | |

Source: U.S. Census of Population, 1970. Prepublication tabulations. Bureau of the Census. U.S. Department of Commerce, 1972.

It is a telling measure of the extent of occupational sex typing that women account for over 80 percent of all workers in nine of the ten leading occupations for women; five are over 95 percent female. And more detailed analysis of specific occupations reveals still further segregation: for example, assemblers in the automotive industry are usually male, while in the lower-paid electronics industry they are predominantly female.

Narrowing the scope still further, the internal labor market of a given firm is often highly sex-segregated. In retail department stores, for example, salaried salesclerks are typically female; those who work on salary-plus-commission in the appliance and furniture departments are usually men. That sex typing is often its own excuse is highlighted by the National Manpower Council's splendidly ludicrous finding that in the Midwest "cornhuskers are traditionally women, while trimmers are almost always men. In the Far West cornhuskers are men and trimmers are women."[2]

*Systemic Segregation*

The actions of working women, working men, and employers and the laws of supply and demand all interact to perpetuate the segregated labor market. Despite high unemployment, men are proving far less eager to work as secretaries, cashiers, and nurses than are women to enter traditional male jobs. "Clearly," according to *Women in Industry*, "when an occupation begins to be thought of as women's work, men do not want to be associated with that type of work."[3]

A more substantive reason for such reluctance is that women's jobs pay extremely poorly relative to men's. Last year women working full-time grossed an average of $166 weekly, only 61 percent of the average for men, $272. And, as figure 1 shows, the earnings gap between men and women is steadily widening. In 1955 women earned 64 cents for every dollar earned by men; in 1977 women's earning power had dropped to 58 cents per dollar.

Apparently most jobs in which women predominate pay poorly (1) because the narrow range of female occupations makes for an oversupply of labor in any given occupation, depressing wages, and (2) precisely because women hold them. According to Eleanor Holmes Norton, chairperson of the Equal Employment Opportunity Commission, "Many jobs continue to be paid on the basis that they will be filled by women and not on the basis of the skills they require."[4] Studies show that though some of the wage differential is attributable to authentic differences in continuity of work experience, adjusting for such differences still leaves much to be explained. Furthermore, a study using Census Bureau and Social Security Administration records corroborates earlier findings that women receive less return for continuous

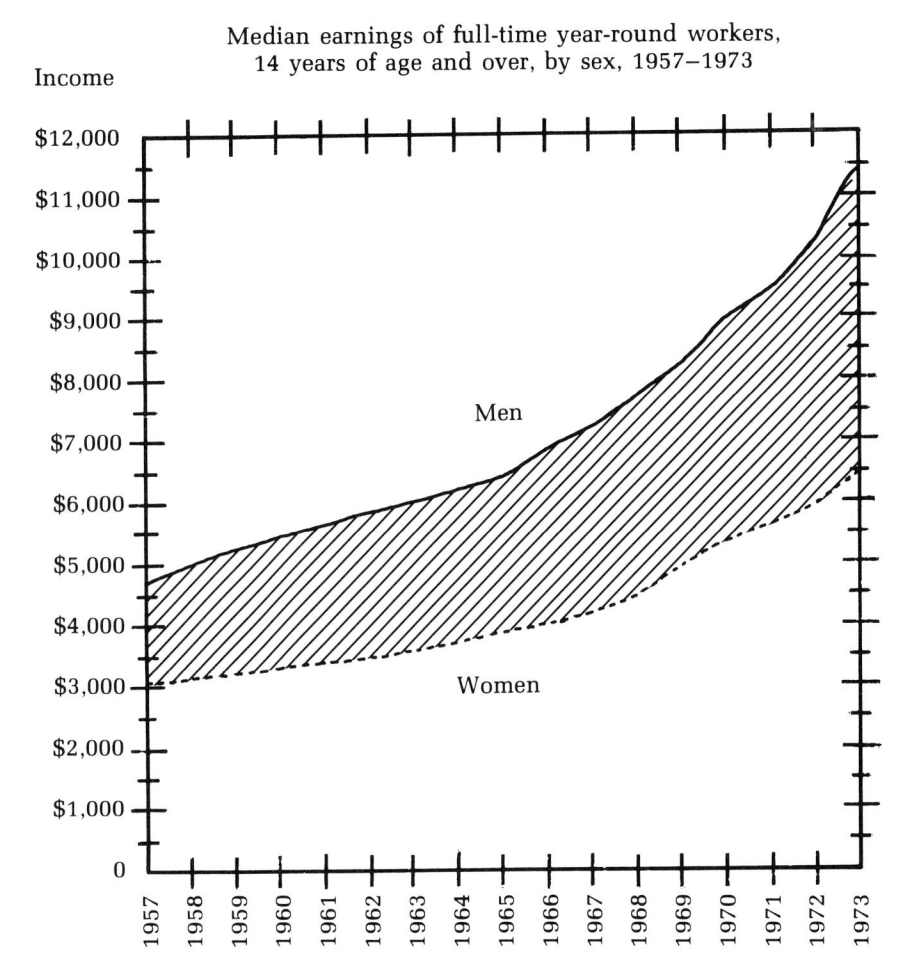

Median earnings of full-time year-round workers, 14 years of age and over, by sex, 1957–1973

**Figure 1**
The Earnings Gap between Women and Men Continues to Widen

Note: Data for 1967–1973 are not strictly comparable with those for prior years, which are for wage and salary income only and do not include earnings of self-employed persons.

Source: *1975 Handbook On Women Workers* (Washington, D.C.: U.S. Department of Labor, Employment Standards Administration, Women's Bureau, 1975): 129; data drawn originally from United States Census.

work experience than do men. As men mature, their earnings rise steeply; women's wage profile is flat. In sum, most of women's wage disadvantage is unexplainable except as systemic discrimination—the kind of discrimination that is hardest to address because of its very pervasiveness.

If discontinuous work patterns help enable employers to underpay women, it should be noted that the process works in reverse as well: low pay and lack of incentives to remain in the work force or with a given employer contribute to high turnover. A recent report in the *Wall Street Journal* suggests that in higher paying management jobs, men's and women's turnover rates are more nearly identical. Motorola reports no difference; at a Chicago bank, the rate is higher for men than for women. Ryder System, a truck-leasing company, reports that among all employees women leave at a higher rate than men, but that among managers at the company headquarters the rate is identical.[5]

*The Pattern of Women's Labor Force Participation*

The typical pattern of women's working lives is to work for a few years, quit to bear and care for children, and eventually reenter the work force (usually when the children are still young) at the same or a lower level. It is quite common for a woman to move in and out of the labor force several times, depending on the number of children and other circumstances.

Working women are more likely than not to be employed part-time and/or less than a full year. The well-heralded figures on women's work force participation rate tend to obscure this fact, since they are based on employment at a given point in time. Largely because they must compromise between their home responsibilities and the requirements of paid employment, the majority of working women work part-time or engage in short periods of employment. And, as Louise Howe points out in her incisive and moving *Pink Collar Workers: Inside the World of Women's Work*, it is precisely the occupations dominated by women that offer opportunities for part-time and intermittent work.

Small firms that rely on female labor, such as restaurants and retail shops, have always hired part-time workers. Hospitals and other health care settings run on variable shifts. It is less well known that both part-time and seasonal work are prevalent and spreading in manufacturing, banking, insurance, utilities, and large-scale retail and wholesale trade. A 1978 survey of over 300 large corporate employers conducted by The Conference Board found that 48 percent of the manufacturers, over 70 percent of the nonmanufacturing companies, and virtually all the banks and utilities employ part-time help.[6] Profitability is undoubtedly a major factor in the spread of part-time work.

Of the surveyed companies' part-time employees, 78 percent are women; in the economy as a whole, two out of three part-time workers are women. Though seasonal work, as defined by the employer, is less widespread (41 percent of the surveyed companies report it), women who need to can and do create their own seasonal work by exercising the right to quit. It is noteworthy, too, that the female-dominated professions—elementary school teaching, nursing, library science, and medical technology—are also characterized by part-time and seasonal work.

*The Costs of Part-Time and Discontinuous Work*

It is no accident that the jobs whose hours are most attractive to women with heavy home responsibilities tend to be far less attractive by any other measure. An occupation that can be abandoned and reentered several years later is likely to offer few opportunities for advancement; in many such occupations, the entry level job is virtually the only job, and there is no route of access to management. As a consequence, pay scales are flat.

It is unsurprising, in this context, that marriage and childbearing increase the likelihood that a woman will experience downward mobility from her first to her latest or last job: of married white women who have had at least one child, 15 percent advanced occupationally and 20 percent retreated. The rest, apparently, experienced no change at all, which may be considered tantamount to downward mobility.[7]

*Employee Benefits and Social Security*

Such jobs also tend to offer few or no benefits, which may be a major reason why they are becoming so much more prevalent. The significance of this situation for women's health and economic security cannot be overstated. A sizeable proportion of American working women are entirely unprotected against the economic effects of illness or injury. A typical example is a divorced woman who supports her children by working as a salesclerk in a department store; if she catches pneumonia or breaks her leg, she is likely to lose her job, lose her income, and be unable to pay her medical bills. Many of the women Howe interviewed for *Pink Collar Workers* reported that they simply try not to think about what would happen if they became too sick to work.

For both married and unmarried women who work part-time or seasonally, lack of access to pension plans can have devastating long-term effects. Three out of four husbands die before their wives, and—as many wives are unaware—the widow may not be covered by her husband's pension. If she has no pension of her own, even despite years of employment, she is likely to retire with very little income.

In sum, many women are seriously disadvantaged by the typical benefit plan's heavy emphasis on conventional full-time, full-year employment. The premium on continuity of employment especially penalizes working mothers. According to The Conference Board's *Women and Employee Benefits*, "There is reluctance to extend life insurance, health coverage, and disability income benefits. . . . These benefits are provided for the part-time work force by 25 to 42 percent of the companies that provide the coverage to full-time people." (These figures are misleading in that they draw on large corporations with unusually extensive benefit plans. Coverage of part-timers is far less commonplace in the economy as a whole.) "Few companies extend any of the benefits package to [the seasonal] workforce."[8]

The Social Security system, based as it is on male employment patterns and the traditional one-earner family, fails to treat women even-handedly. The extreme complexity of Social Security makes an analysis of its inequities beyond the scope of this paper. From the points of view of various categories of working women, however, the situation is as follows. Though required by law to make Social Security payments, a married employed woman must choose between her own retirement pension and half her husband's pension. Because she is likely to have worked part-time and/or discontinuously, she will be better off taking half her husband's benefits—precisely what she would have received had she never worked. Working wives' own benefits are thus in many cases forfeited. A single woman could argue, meanwhile, that she is at a disadvantage relative to married women in that she is offered no such option and must retire on her own benefits—typically far less than a man's even if she worked full-time her entire adult life. A divorced woman who was married less than ten years is entitled to none of her former husband's benefits. The net effect of these policies—in conjunction with women's widespread lack of access to pension plans—is that many American women retire in poverty, which has obvious ramifications for their health in old age.

## Women's Health and Use of Health Care

### Morbidity, Mortality, and Stress

Women and men differ markedly with regard to patterns and rates of illness, longevity, and causes of death. Males' mortality rates are higher at all ages, beginning before birth, and their average life expectancy is currently several years less than women's.

The prevalence of a number of chronic diseases varies considerably with sex. With regard to some diseases, such as atherosclerosis and gout, hormonal and biochemical factors are known to account for much of the difference. Other disorders, such as anemia and gallbladder disease, are related to reproduction. The mechanisms responsible for still other conditions that affect men and women at very different rates, such as diabetes and rheumatoid arthritis, are unknown. According to Lewis and Lewis, "A variety of biologic and hormonal factors are operative, ranging from genetically related deficiencies in immunoglobulin synthesis among males to the effects of hormones on metabolic processes and the sequelae of reproductive functions among females."[9] There is evidence that, in general, women enjoy greater resistance to infectious and degenerative diseases.[10]

Men are more prone to the major life-threatening chronic diseases, such as heart disease, cancer, and cardiovascular disease (see table 2). Women, meanwhile, have higher age-standardized rates of acute conditions, even excluding reproduction-related events, and of nonfatal chronic conditions. Crudely put, the average American man will die at

### Table 2
### Morbidity-Sex Ratios

| Morbidity | Male Rate/Female Rate |
|---|---|
| Chronic conditions* (prevalence) | |
| Emphysema | 3.06 |
| Coronary heart disease | 1.64 |
| Peptic ulcer | 1.61 |
| Hernia | 1.61 |
| Hypertensive heart disease | 0.62 |
| Diabetes | 0.61 |
| Anemia | 0.51 |
| Arthritis | 0.50 |
| Enteritis/colitis | 0.42 |
| Gallbladder disease | 0.31 |
| Varicose veins | 0.23 |
| Acute conditions (incidence) | |
| All | 0.97 |
| Injuries | 1.35 |
| Infections | 0.98 |
| Respiratory conditions | 0.89 |
| Congenital defects* | |
| Color blindness | 12.5 |
| Clubfoot | 2.0 |
| Pyloric stenosis | 5.0 |
| Cleft lip & cleft palate | 2.0 |

*Excludes those with ratios in the range from 0.67 to 1.50 & low prevalence/incidence rates (i.e., uncommon conditions).

Source: Charles E. Lewis and Mary Ann Lewis, "The Potential Impact of Sexual Equality on Health," New England Journal of Medicine 297 (October 20, 1977): 863–869.

Note: Numbers less than 1 represent an excess of the phenomenon among females; the higher the number, the greater the excess among males.

about age 67 of, say, heart disease or cancer; his wife will outlive him by about seven years, perhaps suffering from arthritis or diabetes and occasional short-term illnesses.

Of the fifteen most common causes of death in the United States, men are at greater risk of all but diabetes mellitus. And, as table 3 shows, males' relative disadvantage has increased over time. Though some of the difference is attributable to physiological factors, the belief is widespread among both health professionals and the general public that more males succumb to such diseases because of their greater exposure to risk-enhancing environments. The conventional explanation is that men suffer more stress on the job, while women have been protected from the disease-promoting effects of occupational stress by being predominantly home-bound.

Although exploration of the relationship between job-related stress and specific illnesses is still mostly at the embryonic stage, associations have been demonstrated with regard to several of the diseases to which

**Table 3**
**Mortality-Sex Ratios for the 15 Most Common Causes of Death in the United States**

| Category | Male Rate/Female Rate | | Change in Rate for Entire Population (%) |
|---|---|---|---|
| | 1950 | 1969 | |
| Heart disease | 1.63 | 1.95 | −15 |
| Cancer | 1.08 | 1.42 | +3 |
| Cerebrovascular disease | 1.07 | 1.18 | −23 |
| Accidents | 2.64 | 2.83 | −4 |
| Influenza & pneumonia | 1.39 | 1.64 | −6 |
| Conditions of early infancy | 1.35 | 1.35 | −1 |
| Diabetes mellitus | 0.66 | 0.90 | +1 |
| Arteriosclerosis | 1.29 | 1.20 | −43 |
| Bronchitis, emphysema & asthma | 2.81 | 4.49 | +106 |
| Cirrhosis | 1.96 | 2.04 | +67 |
| Congenital anomalies | 1.13 | 1.13 | −21 |
| Homicide | 3.36 | 1.44 | +59 |
| Nephritis-nephrosis | 1.25 | 1.44 | −76 |
| Peptic ulcer | 4.61 | 2.70 | −28 |
| Suicide | 3.53 | 2.57 | +3 |

Source: Charles E. Lewis and Mary Ann Lewis, "The Potential Impact of Sexual Equality on Health," New England Journal of Medicine 297 (October 20, 1977): 863–869.
Note: Numbers less than 1 represent an excess of the phenomenon among females; the higher the number, the greater the excess among males.

men succumb disproportionately (coronary heart disease, cerebrovascular disease, arteriosclerosis, peptic ulcer). Other major causes of death for men are plainly related to stress by way of voluntary behavior patterns (smoking-related illnesses such as lung cancer, emphysema, and bronchitis; cirrhosis of the liver; homicide, suicide and some accidents).

The relationship between employment and stress on the one hand, and stress and fatal disease on the other, has elicited predictions that female death rates will rise as more women enter the work force, particularly in traditionally male-dominated jobs. There is as yet no evidence to support this contention (mortality rates do not yet reflect the effects of the recent massive influx of women into the labor force). There has been no increase in female death rates relative to male death rates for any illness that could be considered stress-related, with the exception of lung cancer from smoking. Men's and women's death rates for coronary heart disease are both falling and women's are falling faster. Death due to ulcers is also decreasing for both sexes; in this case, men's are declining faster.

The Framingham Heart Study, which followed 900 women aged 45–74 between 1965 and 1973, found that women who worked for pay more than half their adult lives were not significantly more likely to develop heart disease than those who remained at home. Marriage and children, however, apparently increase a woman's risk of heart disease.[11]

Women in the professions and management must cope with the strains of direct competition with men and other women, more-than-full-time jobs, and often residual habits of mind that militate against success, in addition to home responsibilities. On the other hand, professional women often earn enough to buy household services and child care, and report more job satisfaction than less well-educated and well-paid women. It is simply too early to know about the eventual effects of these factors on such women's health. One possibility is that, instead of succumbing to the same diseases that strike their male colleagues, they will experience higher-than-average incidence of the diseases most prevalent among women.

## Women's Use of Health Services

The findings reported above suggest that women are biologically hardier and less at risk of serious illness than men; they are also supposedly protected from exposure to sources of stress. Nevertheless, women consistently visit physicians and use health services more than men, report more physical illness, use more prescription and nonprescription drugs, predominate among psychiatric outpatients, self-report more psychosomatic problems, have higher rates of disability due to acute conditions, and visit physicians more with vague symptoms.

*The Paradox of Illness and Illness Behavior*

What is to be made of the discrepancy between morbidity and use of services? It seems self-apparent that those who are most seriously at risk, most subject to stress, and generally sickest should use health care services most. Thus this anomalous pattern is customarily interpreted to mean that men use health care services more or less appropriately, erring somewhat on the side of underutilization, while women tend toward excessive and hypochondriacal use of care. The argument that high health care costs are in large part attributable to overuse of services tends in turn to promote criticism of women's use of health care.

There is considerable disagreement about the degree to which pregnancy, childbirth, and other reproduction-related conditions account for women's disproportionate use of health services. Some investigators attribute virtually all the male-female differential to this factor; others say it accounts for fractions ranging from approximately one-third to nine-tenths.

Stress appears to be a central factor in various kinds of departure from health. *Webster's New Collegiate Dictionary* defines *stress* as "a physical, chemical, or emotional factor that causes bodily or mental tension and may be a factor in disease causation." Dr. Hans Selye, whose seminal work has contributed greatly to understanding of the etiology of stress-related disease, labels the causative factor a *stressor*; for him the term *stress* applies to the resulting process: "Stress is essentially the rate of all the wear and tear caused by life."[12] This remarkably compendious definition leaves room for all possible causes and makes no distinction whatever between the physical and the emotional.

The prevailing popular understanding of the term, meanwhile, emphasizes external causation. In particular, stress is associated in the popular mind with a complex of circumstances prevalent in certain jobs in which males predominate: pressure to succeed, competition, enforced conformity, deadlines, hostility, rigid hierarchy, and pressure from above are among the factors most commonly associated with stress. Experimental and epidemiological investigations have in turn tended to concentrate on these factors. However, there is nothing inherent in the definition or nature of stress that limits causation to these factors, and self-reported subjective feelings of stress are also strongly associated with other clusters of circumstances.

Unemployment, for example, is highly stressful, especially for women.[13] At-home mothers of young children report considerable distress from constant interruptions, never-completed tasks, lack of variation, economic dependence, and limited adult companionship. Working mothers find it stressful trying to balance their two sets of responsibilities. The "empty-nest syndrome" that afflicts nonemployed mothers whose children have left home is well-documented. But if these situations are genuinely stressful, why is there such a discrepancy between men's and women's vulnerability to stress-related disease?

One possible answer is suggested by asking a further question: what is the precise difference between stress-related illness and psychosomatic illness, which the literature attributes disproportionately to women? *Webster's* defines *psychosomatic* as "of, relating to, or resulting from the interaction and interdependence of psychological and somatic factors." Thus the dictionary definitions of the two terms appear to describe essentially the same process or processes, and differ only in emphasis. While the definition of *psychosomatic* emphasizes the internal process by which psyche and soma interact, the definition of *stress* emphasizes initial external causation and eventual somatic effect. The lack of acknowledgment of external factors in the definition of *psychosomatic* tends to lend to the term a greater aura of craziness and/or invention; common usage ascribes greater legitimacy and severity to stress-related illness than to psychosomatic illness. It is instructive to note the conjunction between value-laden categorization of illness and male-female differences in incidence.

*Possible Protective Effects of Women's Use of Health Care*

To return to the original question, what conclusion ought to be drawn from the inconsistency between patterns of illness and use of health services? The simplest possible answer would be an equation: that women's tendency to seek medical help more readily has a mitigating effect on mortality rates in that it allows for earlier diagnosis and treatment. But this conjecture leaves a great deal unexplained, since what the data show is not that men and women contract the same illnesses and die differentially, but that they tend in general to fall prey to different illnesses.

The differences we have noted in men's and women's physiology, morbidity and mortality patterns, use of health services, occupational patterns, and roles in the family coincide with other differences that may prove pertinent here, namely strikingly different patterns of childhood socialization and of emotional outlets and expressiveness. The tendency of childhood socialization patterns to encourage in girls, and discourage in boys, emotional expressiveness, acknowledgment of individual weaknesses, and preoccupation with subjective feelings has been exhaustively analyzed. It has also been demonstrated that by age 6 little girls already perceive their own health as more precarious and regard health care as more beneficial than do boys of the same age.[14] A study of 5–12-year-old children allowed to initiate their own health care in an elementary school found that girls sought more care than boys, in a proportion similar to that of adults in the general population.[15] Adult women in turn allow themselves more readily than men to pursue medical care with such complaints as chronic fatigue, tension, insomnia, nervousness, digestive problems, and depression. One significant difference between the sexes seems to be how sick one must be before allowing oneself to seek care.

Thus it is plausible that women's greater utilization of health care services is part-and-parcel of a generalized tendency to ventilate rather than ignore emotional distress and strain, and that such care-seeking behavior per se has a protective effect against certain types of severe illness.

It has not yet been demonstrated whether sex-specific behavior patterns have more or less influence than occupational differences on relative morbidity and mortality rates. If behavioral differences indeed prove more influential, it is unlikely that women's vulnerability to stress-related illness will rise significantly as a result of their influx into the work force unless their patterns of care seeking change as well.

Lest this interpretation of women's disproportionate use of health-care services seems excessively benign, it should be pointed out that it also may have as a dark underside the overprescribing and overuse of tranquilizing and mood-altering drugs, and possibly unnecessary medical and surgical procedures as well. But if there is a substantial trade-off effect with fatal illness, women's care-seeking behavior may be seen as both longevity-enhancing and in the long run cost-effective. According to a recent article in the *New England Journal of Medicine*, "the concept of equality need not imply that females change to match a male 'standard.' In contrast, men could benefit enormously if their sex-role changes carried with them some of the protective effects associated with a diminished 'macho' stance. . . . What is the better measure of equality—for women to die like men, or for men to live (a little bit) like women?"[16]

## Women and Disability

Disability may be defined as the conjunction of illness and the illness role, with particular pertinence to eligibility for paid employment. Generally speaking, though the findings of different studies differ, women appear to have higher rates of short-term disability than men.

Several investigators have concluded that sex differences in short-term disability are due less to differences in incidence and severity than to behavioral differences.[17] According to Enterline, "Were it possible to remove the influence of family and other social and cultural factors, females would no doubt have a superior sickness-absence record when compared to males."[18] This statement appears to suggest that the decisive factors are women's exaggerated perceptions of their degree of incapacitation and others' excessive protectiveness. Without disputing the possible influence of such factors, it is interesting to note another interpretation. A large-scale British study of workers incapacitated for paid employment for six months or more by chronic disease found that "women continue to cope with their domestic tasks long after their physical condition has removed them from employment." The investigators postulated that the physicians who certified disability took women's household responsibilities into account, basing their judgments on the patient's capacity to continue paid work on top of unpaid work in the home. Thus, women with heavy household responsibilities may be subject to different criteria of disability than men, certainly a defensible situation on medical grounds.

## Women and Absenteeism

Women are more likely than men to be absent from work (see table 4). Interestingly enough, the differential is greatest (4.9 percent) at ages 25-34 and next highest at 35-44 (3.6 percent); furthermore, female absenteeism is far greater at ages 25-34 than in any other age group except over 65. This pattern does not correspond to the incidence of illness by age, suggesting that a good deal of women's absenteeism, whether attributed to illness or not, is really emergency child care: nearly three-quarters of working women 25-34 have young children. Four times out of five, it is the mother who stays home when a child is sick, while her husband goes to work.[19] As long as employers fail to provide explicitly for paid time off to care for sick children, working mothers have few options. According to The Conference Board's survey of 309 corporations, about 13 percent do provide such time off.[20]

## Effects of Paid Employment on Women's Health

There is no evidence that employment per se—as distinguished from particular hazardous jobs—has a detrimental effect on women's health. On the contrary, Ehrenreich reports that national health surveys taken over the past two decades have found "employed women are less likely [than at-home women] to report having been sick enough to go to bed within the last year, less likely to report chronic conditions such as arthritis, and less likely to complain of miscellaneous 'pains and ailments.' "[21] These findings are particularly intriguing in that they

## Table 4
### Percent of All Wage and Salary Workers on Unscheduled Absence from Work by Sex and Age, May 1976

| Sex and Age | Total Absent Total | Total Absent Illness | Total Absent Other | Absent Part of the Week Total | Absent Part of the Week Illness | Absent Part of the Week Other | Absent the Entire Week Total | Absent the Entire Week Illness | Absent the Entire Week Other |
|---|---|---|---|---|---|---|---|---|---|
| **WOMEN** | | | | | | | | | |
| Total, 16 years and over | 8.6 | 5.1 | 3.4 | 6.0 | 3.4 | 2.6 | 2.5 | 1.7 | 0.8 |
| 16 to 19 | 7.9 | 4.1 | 3.8 | 6.3 | 3.5 | 2.9 | 1.4 | 0.7 | 0.7 |
| 20 to 24 | 8.3 | 5.0 | 3.3 | 6.4 | 4.0 | 2.4 | 1.9 | 1.0 | 0.9 |
| 25 to 34 | 9.7 | 5.6 | 4.1 | 6.4 | 3.7 | 2.7 | 3.3 | 1.8 | 1.4 |
| 35 to 44 | 8.0 | 5.0 | 3.0 | 6.1 | 3.5 | 2.7 | 1.9 | 1.5 | 0.3 |
| 45 to 54 | 8.2 | 4.9 | 3.3 | 5.7 | 2.9 | 2.7 | 2.6 | 2.0 | 0.6 |
| 55 to 64 | 7.9 | 5.0 | 2.9 | 5.1 | 2.8 | 2.3 | 2.8 | 2.2 | 0.6 |
| 65 and over | 10.2 | 7.4 | 3.3 | 3.7 | 2.0 | 2.0 | 6.6 | 5.3 | 1.2 |
| **MEN** | | | | | | | | | |
| Total, 16 years and over | 5.2 | 3.3 | 1.9 | 3.3 | 1.8 | 1.5 | 1.9 | 1.5 | 0.4 |
| 16 to 19 | 6.6 | 3.0 | 3.7 | 5.6 | 2.2 | 3.3 | 1.1 | 0.7 | 0.4 |
| 20 to 24 | 5.7 | 3.2 | 2.5 | 4.3 | 2.2 | 2.1 | 1.5 | 1.0 | 0.5 |
| 25 to 34 | 4.8 | 3.0 | 1.8 | 3.4 | 1.9 | 1.5 | 1.4 | 1.1 | 0.3 |
| 35 to 44 | 4.4 | 2.8 | 1.6 | 2.6 | 1.5 | 1.2 | 1.7 | 1.3 | 0.4 |
| 45 to 54 | 5.2 | 3.5 | 1.7 | 3.0 | 1.7 | 1.2 | 2.2 | 1.8 | 0.4 |
| 55 to 64 | 6.0 | 4.5 | 1.5 | 2.8 | 1.6 | 1.1 | 3.2 | 2.9 | 0.3 |
| 65 and over | 8.5 | 4.2 | 4.2 | 5.0 | 1.0 | 4.0 | 3.5 | 3.3 | 0.2 |

Source: *U.S. Working Women: A Databook* (Washington, D.C.: U.S. Department of Labor, Bureau of Labor Statistics, 1977): 58.
Note: Data exclude agricultural and private household workers and those who held more than one job.

suggest that paid employment may tend to modify women's illness behavior, utilization of services, and morbidity. It should be noted, however, that there are other possible interpretations, among them that employed women are self-selected for health and/or cannot afford to act sick. With regard to stress-related illness in particular, it bears repeating that the Framingham Heart Study found that women who had been employed for more than half their adult lives were not significantly more likely than those who had remained at home to develop heart disease.

There is, however, considerable variation in the relative hazardousness of different kinds of jobs—though not what the conventional wisdom about stressful executive jobs would suggest. The Framingham Heart Study found that women in the traditional female jobs of clerical work and sales are more likely than either blue-collar or professional and business women to develop coronary heart disease. The factors that correlated most closely with heart disease were, interestingly enough, a nonsupportive boss and suppressed hostility; Type A behavior was not found to be a contributing factor. Similarly, a 1977 study by the National Institute of Occupational Safety and Health ranking 130 occupations according to incidence of reported mental illness found nursing and other health-related jobs, waitressing, and clerical work to head the list.[22]

## Hazards of Women's Jobs

Many female occupations are highly hazardous and physically stressful, as table 5 documents. In general, the hazards of women's jobs have received little study. Female-dominated workplaces also tend to be minimally regulated by the Occupational Safety and Health Administration, which concentrates its efforts on major industries and large workplaces. Women thus tend to be less well-protected than men from the effects of workplace hazards. It is noteworthy that many of the women who work in such hazardous settings lack health and disability benefits.

Many women's jobs are also exacting, monotonous, and dead-end. Such jobs take a toll on the women who hold them. (Some men have dull jobs, too, of course, but they pay better and promise wage increases with increasing experience.) As Rosabeth Moss Kanter argues provocatively in *Men and Women of the Corporation*,

> Those whose mobility is limited or blocked can develop a self-image that matches their situation. . . . Textile workers . . . are a good example. A high proportion of the production workers in this industry are women. The jobs characteristically pay low wages and

## Table 5
### Examples of Occupational Exposures in Predominantly Female Jobs

| Occupation | Exposures |
|---|---|
| 1. Textile and Related Operatives | |
| a. Textile operatives | raw cotton dust, noise, synthetic fiber dusts, formaldehyde, heat, dyes, flame retardants, asbestos |
| b. Sewers and stitchers | cotton and synthetic fiber dusts, noise, formaldehyde, organic solvents, flame retardants, asbestos |
| c. Upholsterers | same as above |
| (Some specific chemicals encountered in the above occupations are: benzene, toluene, trichloroethylene, perchloroethylene, chloroprene, styrene, carbon disulfide.) | |
| 2. Hospital/Health Personnel | |
| a. Registered nurses, aides, orderlies | anesthetic gases, ethylene oxide, x-ray radiation, alcohol, infectious diseases, puncture wounds |
| b. Dental hygienists | x-ray radiation, mercury, ultrasonic noise, anesthetic gases |
| c. Laboratory workers (clinical and research) | wide variety of toxic chemicals, including carcinogens, mutagens and teratogens, x-ray radiation |
| 3. Electronics Assemblers | lead, tin, antimony, trichloroethylene, methylene chloride, epoxy resins, methyl ethyl ketone |
| 4. Hairdressers and Cosmetologists | hair spray resins (polyvinyl pyrolidone), aerosol propellants (freons), halogenated hydrocarbons, hair dyes, solvents of nail polish, benzyl alcohol, ethyl alcohol, acetone |
| 5. Cleaning Personnel | |
| a. Launderers | soaps, detergents, enzymes, heat, humidity, industrially contaminated clothing |
| b. Dry cleaners | perchloroethylene, trichloroethylene, stoddard solvent (naphtha), benzene, industrially contaminated clothing |
| 6. Photographic Processors | caustics, iron salts, mercuric chloride, bromides, iodides, pyrogallic acid, and silver nitrate |
| 7. Plastic Fabricators | acrylonitrile, phenol-formaldehydes, urea-formaldehydes, hexamethylene-tetramine, acids, alkalies, peroxide, vinyl chloride, polystyrene, vinylidene chloride |

**Table 5** (*Continued*)
**Examples of Occupational Exposures in Predominantly Female Jobs**

| Occupation | Exposures |
|---|---|
| 8. Domestics | solvents, hydrocarbons, soaps, detergents, bleaches, alkalies |
| 9. Transportation Operatives | carbon monoxide, polynuclear aromatics, lead and other combustion products of gasoline, vibration, physical stresses |
| 10. Sign Painters and Letterers | lead oxide, lead chromate pigments, epichlorohydrin, titanium dioxide, trace metals, xylene, toluene |
| 11. Clerical Personnel | physical stresses, poor illumination, trichloroethylene, carbon tetrachloride and various other cleaners, asbestos in air conditioning |
| 12. Opticians and Lens Grinders | coal tar pitch volatiles, iron oxide dust solvents, hydrocarbons |
| 13. Printing Operatives | ink mists, 2-nitropropane, methanol carbon tetrachloride, methylene chloride, lead, noise, hydrocarbon solvents, trichloroethylene, toluene, benzene, trace metals |

Source: American College of Obstetricians and Gynecologists, *Guidelines on Pregnancy and Work* (Washington, D.C.: U.S. Department of Health, Education, and Welfare, Public Health Service, Center for Disease Control, National Institute for Occupational Safety and Health, 1977): 64–66.

offer little freedom, and women tend to be concentrated especially in low-involvement jobs. . . . There are very limited opportunities for advancement—few skilled jobs, a narrow wage spread, and a limited occupational ladder. Yet . . . the women's self-image fits the job. They have low estimates of their own abilities and possibilities.[23]

A study undertaken in 1978 by the National Commission on Working Women, a branch of the National Manpower Institute, surveyed 150,000 employed women on their work-related problems and attitudes toward their jobs. Financed by several large corporations and the United Auto Workers, the survey is the largest of its kind ever conducted. According to a *Boston Globe* report on the study, "America's average working woman describes herself as frustrated, working in a dead-end job with no chance in sight for advancement or training opportunities. She is underpaid, underutilized and afforded little or no respect for the work she contributes. . . . 55 percent of the professional women surveyed and 50 percent of clerical, sales, service, and blue-collar workers say they have no leisure time."[24] The implications for mental health are self-apparent, if not precisely measurable.

## The Legal and Regulatory Context

The workplace offers unique challenges to the interpretation of antidiscrimination law in that authentic differences between women and men that are immaterial in other settings may have, or appear to have, considerable pertinence at work. It is a matter of concern in various kinds of jobs that the sexes are, if equal, not identical: that women can conceive and bear children, that men are more susceptible to chemically induced sterility, that men's and women's morbidity patterns are different, and/or that the sexes differ in various types of strength and endurance. Before examining a series of situations in which genuine differences between the sexes are at issue, let us review the legal constraints on employers and the limitations of protective legislation.

Federal law unequivocally prohibits sex discrimination in hiring and firing, wages and salaries, benefits, promotions, layoffs, training, and other conditions of employment. There are few exemptions from coverage by Title VII of the 1964 Civil Rights Act; all private employers of fifteen or more persons are obliged to comply. Exceptions are provided for only when sex is a bona fide occupational qualification, and this clause has been interpreted very narrowly—the Department of Labor offers as examples the jobs of actor and wet nurse. The guidelines issued by the Equal Employment Opportunity Commission, which administers Title VII, specify that hiring and other decisions cannot be based on assumptions about the characteristics of women in general or on customers' preferences for one sex over the other. Courts have ruled that, in light of Title VII, employers may not assign light work to women and heavy work to men. A Supreme Court decision has held that discrimination need not be intentional to be unlawful.

The Equal Pay Act of 1963, considerably more limited in scope, prohibits employers from paying women less than men for jobs that require equal skill, effort, and responsibility and are performed under similar working conditions. Pay differentials based on seniority, a merit system, volume of piecework, or any standard other than sex are permitted. In interpreting this law, the Supreme Court has declared that jobs need only be "substantially equal," not identical, to qualify for equal pay.

## LEGISLATION AFFECTING THE RIGHTS OF WOMEN WORKERS

| U.S. Constitutional Amendments | Legislation | Administering Agency |
|---|---|---|
| Article XIV: Section I: "All persons born or naturalized in the United States and subject to the jurisdiction thereof, are citizens of the United States and of the State wherein they reside. No State shall make or enforce any law which shall abridge the privilege or immunities of citizens of the United States; nor shall any State deprive any person of life, liberty or property without the due process of law; nor deny to any person within its jurisdiction the equal protection of the laws." (The Fifth Amendment provides the same protections as regards the federal government.) | Civil Rights Act of 1964, Title VII: guarantees the rights to employment without sex, race, color, creed, religion, or national origin discrimination | Equal Employment Opportunity Commission |
| | Equal Employment Opportunity Act of 1972: amends and broadens Title VII | |
| | Pregnancy Disability Act of 1978: requires employers to treat pregnancy-related absences like absences for other disabilities | |
| | Fair Labor Standards Act of 1938: establishes minimum wage, overtime, etc. | Wage and Hour Division, Department of Labor |
| | Equal Pay Act of 1963: most recent amendment to the Fair Labor Standards Act | |
| | Occupational Safety and Health Act of 1970: guarantees a safe and healthful workplace to all workers | Occupational Safety and Health Administration, Department of Labor |
| | State Fair Employment Practices Statutes | Appropriate state agency |

Source: Adapted from Jeanne M. Stellman, *Women's Work, Women's Health: Myths and Realities* (New York: Pantheon Books, 1977): table 26, p. 191.

In finding the jobs of nurses' aide and orderly at a hospital equal, the Fourth Circuit Court of Appeals stated that higher pay for males cannot be justified on the grounds of extra tasks if (1) some men receive the higher rate without doing extra work; (2) women also perform comparable extra tasks; (3) qualified female employees are not eligible to do the extra work; (4) the extra tasks consume little time and are of peripheral importance; and/or (5) a third group of employees who perform the extra tasks as their primary job are paid less than the male employees in question (*Brennan v. Prince William Hospital*, 503 F.2d 282). In another case, the Supreme Court held that men who work the night shift cannot be paid more than women who do the same work on the day shift on the grounds of dissimilar working conditions.

Violations of the Equal Pay Act have resulted in some large awards of back wages to female employees, and Title VII has had similar effectiveness. Nevertheless, federal law has serious limitations as a mechanism for promoting equality of the sexes in the labor market. The problem is not that the laws themselves were inadequately framed; they go about as far as they can. But such laws must of their nature focus on concrete discriminatory acts and policies, and discrimination can only be demonstrated in situations of comparability.

If, for example, a company employs both men and women as packers but pays the men more, it is violating the Equal Pay Act. If the company hires only women as stackers and only men as packers, it is violating Title VII; if the two jobs are substantially equal and packers are paid more, it is in violation of the Equal Pay Act as well.

But what about the company secretaries and typists? Female secretaries are probably paid no less than male secretaries, because there are no male secretaries. Nor are there usually men with another job title doing work substantially equal to that of a secretary. The employer cannot usually be faulted for failing to hire men as secretaries; it is likely that none applied.

If, in this hypothetical company, the job of secretary pays a decent salary, provides for substantial salary increases with seniority, entails well-defined responsibilities, and offers opportunities for advancement, there may be no problem. But if there is a problem—if the secretarial salary scale is relatively flat, say, or if secretaries' salaries depend on their bosses' whims, or if secretarial jobs lead nowhere—antidiscrimination law is not a ready remedy.

In other words, federal antidiscrimination law does not protect women from unfavorable working conditions per se; it only protects them from worse working conditions than male counterparts with the same employer, if there are any. If there is no "control group" of comparable men, discrimination cannot be demonstrated. It is safe to say that well over half of American working women have virtually no direct male counterparts. Of the ten occupations employing the most women, secretaries, typists, and registered nurses are almost exclusively female throughout the nation, and all the others except elementary school teacher are likely in any given workplace to be performed exclusively by women. Nor is the law well equipped to address certain kinds of sex-neutral practices that affect women disproportionately, such as the denial of fringe benefits to part-time employees.

This is by no means to say that equal opportunity law is a paper tiger. Many employers have felt its bite, and working women benefit extensively from its protection. But sex segregation in the job market is so pervasive and so multiply caused that many of its most overt manifestations cannot be readily corrected by acts of law.

## Hazards Facing Women in Traditionally Male Jobs

Women who enter untraditional, physically demanding occupations—machinists, construction workers, telephone-line installers, firefighters, laborers, and the like—face some unique problems and hazards. Though, as one such woman acknowledged, "it's no secret the average man is stronger than the average woman," women have demonstrated—most notably in factories during World War II—the capacity to perform skilled and taxing physical work. Self-selection appears to function relatively efficiently; preemployment testing may justifiably be used in some situations if the test is genuinely pertinent to the demands of the job, unbiased, and administered to men as well.

Because women tend to be less familiar than men with using tools, manipulating equipment, and ways of applying their strength to best advantage, a number of employers' experience shows that training periods may need to be longer, more thorough, and/or more self-paced than is customary.

A more persistent problem is that every aspect of the physical environment in such jobs tends to be designed for the average male. Thus, tools may be too large, worktables too high, control switches out of reach, and the like. Safety equipment and appropriate workclothes and shoes may be ill-fitting or unavailable. When such situations are not corrected and women's accident or turnover rates exceed men's, the tendency still prevails among employers to blame female weakness—a tendency that represents a further pressure on women in untraditional jobs.

Bell System's experience is particularly instructive. Prodded by the federal government, the company responded to women employees' difficulties by lengthening the training program, substituting light fiberglass ladders for wooden ones, lowering the fulcrum used to swing a ladder onto the side of a truck, and other such minor adjustments. As a result, women's turnover and accident rates dropped. Small companies that do not design and manufacture their own equipment may find such measures more problematic.

OSHA's safety regulations, too, are based on the average male, which has the effect of protecting women less well on the job. If they persist, such problems appear to have considerable potential for redress through the courts and/or the Equal Employment Opportunity Commission.

## Pregnancy and Employment

Both the accomplishments and the limitations of federal antidiscrimination legislation with regard to working women are well illustrated by the amendment to Title VII prohibiting discrimination on grounds of pregnancy, which took effect in 1979. The law prohibits employers from discriminating against pregnant workers in any area of employment, including hiring, promotion, job security, seniority, termination, and benefit programs.

The effect of the law will clearly be broadest and most immediate on benefits, where compliance is a matter of across-the-board policy rather than responses to individual cases in which extenuating circumstances can be invoked. The basic operating principle of the new law with regard to benefits—health insurance, disability insurance, and sick leave—is that the employer must treat pregnancy-related disability as any other disability is treated; thus coverage will vary according to company policy.

Pregnancy per se is not a disability; whether and for how long a woman continues working is to be decided on the basis of the recommendation of the woman's physician, and the employer is required to provide benefits only while the woman is medically unable to work. Most women who have a normal pregnancy and delivery are medically able to continue working until labor begins and to return to work about six weeks after giving birth; companies that offer disability insurance typically provide for longer disabilities, usually 15–26 weeks.

To guide physicians in determining whether a particular woman should continue to work and when she can return to work, the American College of Obstetricians and Gynecologists recently issued a set of guidelines commissioned by the National Institute of Occupational Safety and Health. The guidelines' basic premise is that "a normal woman with a normal pregnancy and a normal fetus in a job presenting no greater potential hazards than those encountered in normal daily life in the community may continue to work without interruption until the onset of labor, and may resume working several weeks after an uncomplicated delivery."[25]

The guidelines specify three categories of pregnancy-related disability: that related to the pregnancy itself "as occurs in labor and delivery"; that related to complications, including excess fatigue; and that related to job exposures, such as toxins or abnormal physical stress. The physician is not empowered to determine whether a woman is eligible for disability benefits; he or she is making recommendations for use by the employer in determining disability. Four possible recommendations are specified: the woman may continue to work as before; she may continue to work but a modification of her job or environment is desirable; such a modification is essential if she is to work; or the woman should not work. Figure 2 illustrates the decision-making procedure recommended to physicians by the ACOG guidelines.

It appears likely that disputes will arise over disability related to job exposures. Let us assume that a woman's physician finds that she is physically capable of working but that her job is hazardous to her pregnancy, and thus recommends that she continue to work only if she can be transferred to a safer job. The employer may reply that no such job is available. If the woman then stops working, the employer may in turn refuse her disability benefits on the grounds that she is not medically disabled.

The Boston office of the Equal Employment Opportunity Commission, contacted by telephone, stated that in such a circumstance the operative principle is comparability; that is, a firm that has previously granted a transfer to a male employee who developed, for example, asthma, must do the same for a pregnant employee. Though the protective capacity of this principle has not been tested, it bears repeating that many jobs hazardous to pregnancy are in occupations so female-dominated that they are unlikely to offer such precedents.

The maternity law will probably have less substantial effects in areas other than benefits, since its applicability will arise intermittently, comparability cannot usually be invoked, and violations will be harder to prove. A pregnant woman who is turned down for a job will typically have a harder time proving her case—that pregnancy is the reason for her rejection—than will an employed pregnant woman who is denied benefits due her. According to Noreen Connell, chairperson of the board of the New York Chapter of the National Organization for Women, "Discrimination toward the pregnant woman is still a No. 1 problem. They notify their employer that they're pregnant, and all of a sudden the employer says you're coming in late, or your productivity is low, or there's a layoff. Even though it's totally against the law, women are still getting fired for getting pregnant."[26]

**Figure 2**
Recommended Procedure for Medical Assessment of a Pregnant Woman's Fitness to Work

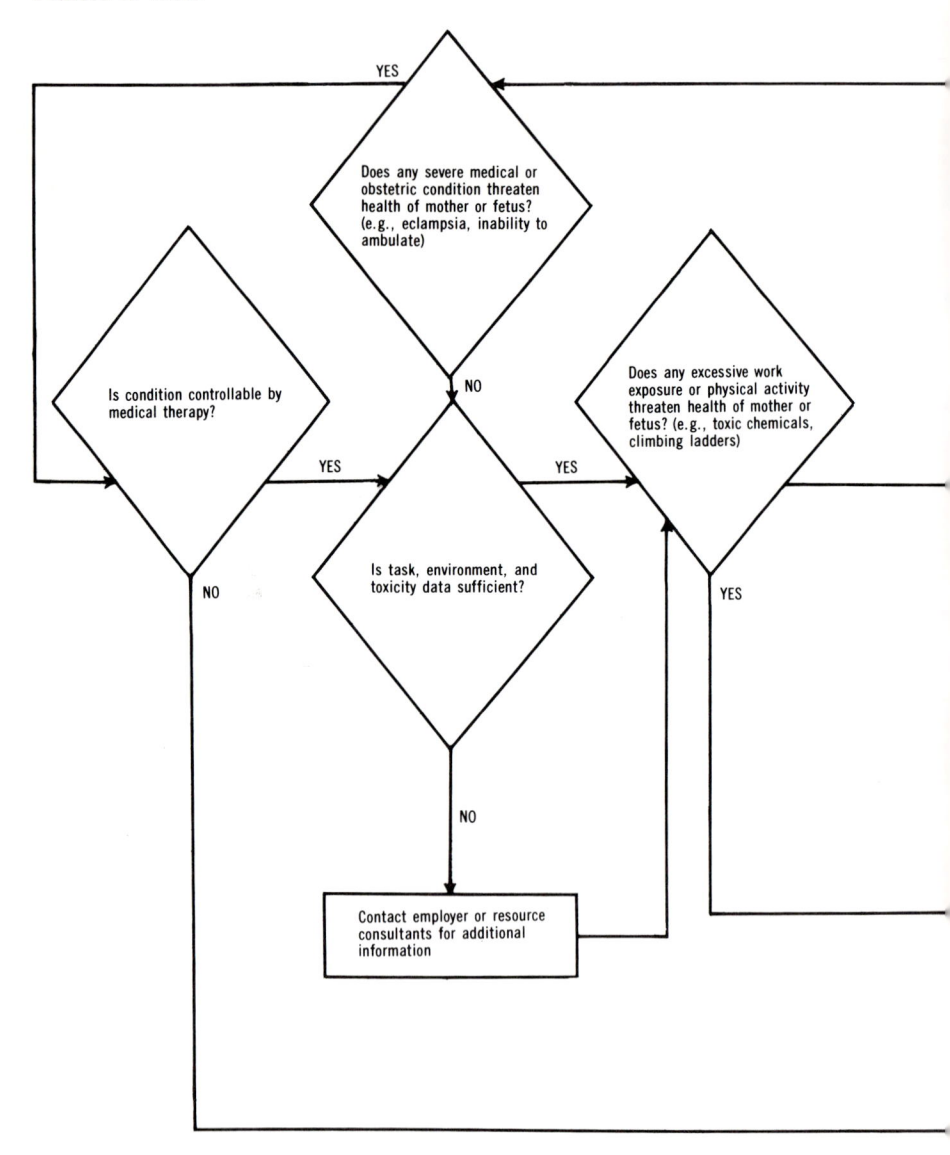

Source: American College of Obstetricians and Gynecologists, *Guidelines on Pregnancy and Work* (Washington, D.C.: U.S. Department of Health, Education, and Welfare, Public Health Service, Center for Disease Control, National Institute for Occupational Safety and Health, 1977): 14.

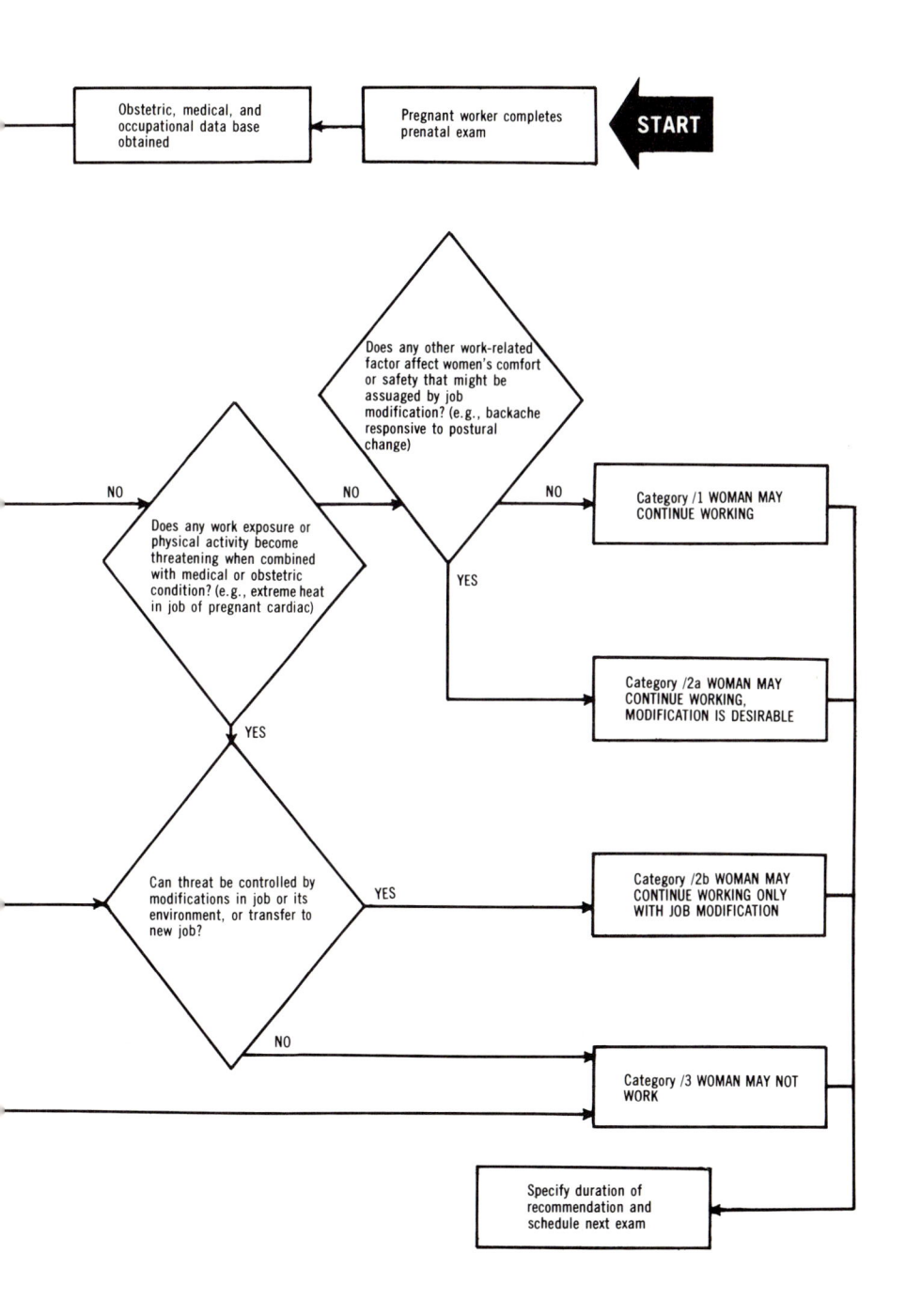

## Overview: The Health of Working Women

**START** → Pregnant worker completes prenatal exam → Obstetric, medical, and occupational data base obtained

**Does any work exposure or physical activity become threatening when combined with medical or obstetric condition? (e.g., extreme heat in job of pregnant cardiac)**
- NO → **Does any other work-related factor affect women's comfort or safety that might be assuaged by job modification? (e.g., backache responsive to postural change)**
  - NO → **Category /1 WOMAN MAY CONTINUE WORKING**
  - YES → **Category /2a WOMAN MAY CONTINUE WORKING, MODIFICATION IS DESIRABLE**
- YES → **Can threat be controlled by modifications in job or its environment, or transfer to new job?**
  - YES → **Category /2b WOMAN MAY CONTINUE WORKING ONLY WITH JOB MODIFICATION**
  - NO → **Category /3 WOMAN MAY NOT WORK**

→ Specify duration of recommendation and schedule next exam

From the vantage point of working women, the major loopholes in this and other protective laws are the eligibility requirements. In order to qualify, a woman must work for a firm with more than fifteen employees that already provides benefits. These requirements shut out most waitresses, beauticians, private household workers, secretaries and typists in small firms, many salesclerks and cashiers—in other words, those occupations that account for most working women. Furthermore, a woman who has worked for her present employer for less than two years, works fewer than twenty weeks a year, or works part-time need not be covered; as we have seen, these requirements render far more women ineligible.

## Reproductive Hazards in the Workplace

Let us look next at a highly inflammatory issue that appears to bring antidiscrimination law into conflict with another piece of landmark protective legislation, the Occupational Safety and Health Act of 1970. Whether viewed medically, legally, politically, emotionally, or from virtually any other vantage point, the most acutely serious issue employed women face today is exposure to fetotoxic substances—substances that can cause death, birth defects, and susceptibility to cancer and other diseases in unborn children.

A number of industrial firms have recently adopted policies prohibiting all women of childbearing age from jobs that would expose them to substances hazardous to unborn children. American Cyanamid, for example, has shifted all women under the age of 50 out of the pigment division of its West Virginia plant, where they were exposed to lead, and subsequently extended the policy to nine other plants throughout the United States. Olin Corporation does not hire women at its ammunition plants, where benzene is used, or at factories where carbon disulfide is used in the manufacture of cellophane. Allied Chemical laid off women packagers at an Illinois plant where they were exposed to a substance called Fluorocarbon 22. Comparable policies have been adopted by General Motors, Exxon, Monsanto, DuPont, Eastman Kodak, Firestone Tire and Rubber, and a number of smaller firms.[27]

Some of the women affected have been offered transfers to janitorial jobs that pay less, provide no opportunities for overtime, and involve loss of seniority. Many have been fired. Only a very few have been transferred at no loss of wages or seniority. The number of women directly affected is by no means small, especially taking into account all those who would otherwise be eligible for such jobs.

Faced with loss of their jobs, some women have reacted to such policies by having themselves sterilized. Among them are five women at American Cyanamid's plant in Willow Island, West Virginia, a depressed area where unemployment is high and few employers pay well; their union, the Oil, Chemical, and Atomic Workers, is submitting the matter to arbitration. After two employees of Allied Chemical underwent sterilization, it was decided that the substance in question, Fluorocarbon 22, was not after all hazardous to the fetus at the levels encountered in the plant. The International Chemical Workers Union recently negotiated an undisclosed cash settlement with Allied Chemical on behalf of these two and three other women who had been fired.

## Fetotoxicity, Teratogenesis, and Mutagenesis

A number of substances manufactured or used in industry and in laboratories are known to harm the human fetus. It has been known since the turn of the century, for example, that women working with lead suffer abnormally high rates of miscarriage and stillbirth; animal studies suggest that lead can also cause birth defects, learning impairment, faulty growth, and nervous disorders. Anesthetic gases and vapors encountered by hospital operating room personnel are known to cause unusually high rates of miscarriage and birth defects. There is evidence that vinyl chloride, used in the production of plastics, can cause cancer in the offspring of exposed workers. Organic solvents appear to increase miscarriage rates and possibly to produce spinal birth defects in children of exposed mothers. Other implicated substances include, but are not limited to, x-rays, carbon monoxide, aniline dyes, formaldehyde, estrogens, pesticides of many types, pharmaceuticals, mercury, carbon disulfide, and polychlorinated biphenyls (PCBs).

Exposure to teratogenic substances can have a variety of disastrous effects, including failure to conceive, miscarriage, stillbirth, and both overt and latent defects. Figure 3 is a partial inventory of occupational exposures and their actual or potential reproductive or systemic effects. It is usually unclear whether a particular outcome is the result of a mutation, the alteration of the genetic material itself (the genes and chromosomes). Mutations of genetic material are permanent; that is, they can continue to affect succeeding generations in perpetuity. Furthermore, mutations may occur at any age, both prenatally and after birth. In other words, the developing fetus is vulnerable to mutagenic agents and so are the sperm and egg cells of adult men and women.

Generally speaking, the fetus is vulnerable to the most severe damage during the first trimester, or first three months, of gestation, when the organs are forming. A mutation or developmental defect that occurs during this period may result in the malformation of one or more organs. After about the eighth week, when the fetus begins to grow rapidly, an environmental insult can retard or halt growth of particular organs or organ systems. "Certain exposures early in pregnancy are followed by miscarriage, later exposures by teratogenesis and still later exposures by malignant degeneration."[28]

One might assume that the effects of a potent teratogen would be unmistakable, as in the case of the thousands of defective babies whose mothers took thalidomide. But the variety of possible outcomes, as well as subtlety and/or delay in the manifestation of some abnormalities, can effectively obscure a pattern of damage. In her admirable and indispensable *Women's Work, Women's Health*, Jeanne Stellman illustrates this point with a forceful hypothetical example:

> Let us assume that a female hairdresser who inhaled six cans of vinyl-chloride-propelled aerosol hairspray vapors each working day produced defective offspring. . . . However, the defects were not easily recognizable traits such as harelip. Instead, the mutation resulted in a subtle biochemical functional disorder leading to a high risk of developing leukemia. If one of her offspring did develop leukemia, that case of leukemia would be just one among thousands, since leukemia is not an exceptionally rare disease and its relationship to other environmental factors is not understood. . . . It is easy to see how such an effect could remain undiscovered, hidden by a general prevalence of the disease in people with no history of parental exposure to large doses of aerosol vapors. If there were thousands of people exposed to the spray and hence thousands of excess cases of leukemia in their offspring, *and* if astute medical practitioners took the appropriate history of parental occupational exposures, *and* if all the data were pooled and analyzed, then *perhaps* we could make an association of cause and effect.[29]

Furthermore, most birth defects cannot be positively attributed to a single cause. Current scientific opinion attributes only about one-quarter of all birth defects to genetic abnormalities and the remainder to complex interactions between environmental insults and genetic susceptibilities. But understanding of the nature of such interactions is still very primitive.

Experimental investigations of the nature and effects of occupational toxins are not routinely undertaken. The National Institute of Occupational Safety and Health (NIOSH), the research arm of the Occupational Safety and Health Administration (OSHA), largely limits its testing to direct physiological reactions, such as skin rashes and

---

**Figure 3 (*facing page*)**
Partial Inventory of Reproductive Toxins and Effects

Source: American College of Obstetricians and Gynecologists, *Guidelines on Pregnancy and Work* (Washington, D.C.: U.S. Department of Health, Education, and Welfare, Public Health Service, Center for Disease Control, National Institute for Occupational Safety and Health, 1977): 16.

| AGENTS | DEFINITIVE SYSTEMIC TOXICITY (Neurologic, Hepatic, Renal, Hematologic, Cardiovascular, Pulmonary) | SPECIAL EFFECTS | SUSPECTED REPRODUCTIVE EFFECTS (Carcinogenesis, Reduced Fertility, Spontaneous Abortion, Mutagenesis, Teratogenesis) | SUGGESTED BIOLOGICAL TESTING | AIR STANDARDS OSHA (existing) | AIR STANDARDS NIOSH (proposed) |
|---|---|---|---|---|---|---|
| **Heavy metals** | | | | | | |
| Cadmium | • • • • • | | • • ○ • | Urine cadmium; Quant. low molecular weight proteins | fume 0.1 mg/M³ dust 0.2 mg/M³ | 40 µg/M³ |
| Lead | • • • | | ○ • • | Blood lead··; Blood zinc protoporphyrin; Urine ALA; Urine coproporphyrin | inorganic 0.2 mg/M³ (Proposed 0.1 mg/M³) | inorganic 0.1 mg/M³ and Blood Lead 60µg/100gms |
| Mercury | • • | | • • | Blood mercury; Urine mercury | inorganic 0.1 mg/M³ organic 0.01 mg/M³ | inorganic 0.05 mg/M³ |
| **Organic solvents** | | | | | | |
| Benzene (benzol) | • • • | | • • | Urine phenols; CBC | 10 ppm (emergency proposal: 1 ppm) | 1 ppm |
| **Halogenated hydrocarbons** | | | | | | |
| 2 chlorobutadiene (chloroprene) | • • • • | | • ○ • • | Liver function test | 25 ppm | 1 ppm |
| Dibromochloropropane | • • | | • ○ | Sperm count; Serum testosterone | 10 ppb (emergency proposed) | 10 ppb |
| Epichlorohydrin | • • • | | • | Liver function test | 20 mg/M³ | 2 mg/M³ |
| Ethylene dibromide | • • | | • ○ | | 20 ppm | 1 mg/M³ |
| Polychlorinated biphenyls (PCB's) | • • • | Chloracne | • • • | Blood analysis; Adipose tissue; Serum transaminase | Compounds with 42% chlorine 1 mg/M³ 54% chlorine 0.5 mg/M³ | 1 µg/M³ |
| Tetrachloroethylene (Perchloroethylene) | • • • | | • • | | 100 ppm | 50 ppm |
| Vinyl chloride | • • • | Acrosteolysis | • • | Liver function test | 1 ppm | 1 ppm |
| **Hypoxic agents** | | | | | | |
| Carbon monoxide | • • • | | • | Carboxy hemoglobin | 50 ppm | 35 ppm |
| **Anesthetic gases** | | | | | | |
| Halogenated gases e.g. halothane methoxy fluorane | • • | | • • • • • | | not specified | Halogenated anesthetics 2 ppm based on weight of specific gas sampled not >1 hour |
| **Pesticides** | | | | | | |
| Carbaryl | • | | • | | 5 mg/M³ | 5 mg/M³ |
| Chlorinated hydrocarbons (e.g. chlordane) | • | | • | Adipose tissue analysis; Blood analysis | varies with specific compounds e.g. Chlordane 0.5 mg/M³ | |
| Chlordecone (kepone) | • • | Pleuritic and joint pains | • ○ | Blood analysis | emergency standard 1 µg/M³ | 1 µg/M³ |
| **Estrogenic compounds** | | | | | | |
| Diethylstilbestrol | • | | • • • | Blood analysis | not specified | not specified |
| **Ionizing radiation (Whole body)** | | | | | | |
| X-rays and gamma rays | • | Gastro-intestinal disorders | • • • • • | Personal film badge dosimetry; Thermoluminscent dosimetry | NCRP recommendation 1.25 rad/quarter, 5 rad/year Pregnancy: 0.5 rem/full pregnancy | |
| **Miscellaneous substances** | | | | | | |
| Carbon disulfide | • • | Retinopathy | • • | Urine iodine-azide test | 20 ppm | 3 mg/M³ |
| Ethylene Oxide | • • | | • | CBC | 50 ppm | 50 ppm |

• Animal and/or human data
· Time weighted average 40-hr. week, 8-hr. day (OSHA), 10-hr. day (NIOSH).
·· In pregnancy, blood lead less than 40 µg/100 gms is suggested.
○ Evidence only male infertility; no data on females

poisoning. Though it is known that substances with minimal direct effects may have long-term toxic effects, NIOSH does not ordinarily investigate such effects, largely for reasons of cost, manpower, and feasibility. Less than 1 percent of the more than 16,000 chemicals in NIOSH's *Registry of Toxic Effects of Chemical Substances* have been tested for mutagenic effects. In setting standards of occupational exposure, OSHA in turn does not ordinarily consider possible teratogenic or carcinogenic effects, nor the synergistic (combined) effects of mixtures of chemicals.

Thus, with regard to most known and suspected industrial toxins, no one knows with certainty what level of exposure, if any, is safe for the fetus—or, for that matter, the adult female or male.

## The Premises of the Debate

Feeling runs very high on all sides of this incendiary issue. The firms in question argue that they are not discriminating against women but protecting unborn children. As one corporate health officer quoted in the *Wall Street Journal* put it, "We don't allow children in the workplace, and we shouldn't allow the fetus in the workplace."[30] Women who have lost their jobs, union representatives, and others argue in response that workplaces should be made safe for all who enter them, including the fetus. Acknowledging that a hazard-free workplace is a long-term goal not amenable to immediate implementation, some have proposed that in the meantime pregnant factory workers be transferred to safe jobs, at no loss of salary or seniority, for the duration of pregnancy and lactation. Before examining these and other alternatives, let us reconsider the premises of the debate.

The publicity and emotion aroused by these events tend to reinforce two inaccurate impressions: that the fetus alone is at risk; and that keeping prospective mothers out of toxic workplaces effectively eliminates such risk. In fact, (1) substances that cause fetal death and genetic mutations can do so through the father as well; according to the ACOG's *Guidelines on Pregnancy and Work*, "Many of these adverse effects are the result of the genetic effects of occupational exposures of men prior to conception."[31] Furthermore, (2) males' reproductive and sexual capacities are uniquely vulnerable to certain toxic substances encountered in the workplace; and (3) evidence is accumulating that most substances that cause mutations can also cause cancer.[32] It appears, in general, that a toxin encountered in the workplace is likely to have several possible varieties of ill effect and to harm more than one subset of the population. Furthermore, the nature of mutagenesis requires that the potential father, the potential mother, and the fetus be regarded as an interrelated system from which no single member can be separated out as bearing the burden of risk.

Exposure to anesthetic gases, for example, has been demonstrated to cause significantly increased rates of miscarriage and birth defects among pregnant operating room personnel and the wives of exposed males. Exposed women run an increased risk of cancer and kidney and liver disease; it is unclear whether males are subject to increased cancer, but they do suffer excess liver disease.

Exposure to vinyl chloride has been associated with teratogenic effects through the mother, mutagenic effects through the father, chromosome aberrations (reported by studies in four countries), elevated miscarriage and stillbirth rates among the wives of exposed males, and markedly increased risk of angiosarcoma of the liver. Recent studies also suggest an increased risk of lung cancer, cancer of the blood-forming tissues, and cancer of the brain and central nervous system.

Lead is associated with low sperm counts, decreased sex drive, and atrophy of the testicles in exposed males; impotence and a decrease in libido have been reported in association with manganese; a high percentage of males exposed to kepone have suffered sterility. Stellman cites numerous further examples.[33]

Thus, the prevailing policy of "protective discrimination" discriminates against women in terms of employment and against men in terms of health hazards. It also fails to achieve its stated intention, which is to protect the fetus. Let us examine the alternatives to it that have been proposed in public debate. As we shall see, they too appear to have serious shortcomings.

## Alternatives to "Protective Discrimination"

Refusing to hire women for certain types of jobs, whether such a policy is intended benignly, protectively, self-protectively, or maliciously, is illegal discrimination—a violation of Title VII. Furthermore, such policies must of their nature discriminate against all women, not just pregnant or fertile women or women actively trying to become pregnant, since it is objectively impossible to distinguish among them without grossly invading privacy. Though there is only incidental evidence of firms' overtly encouraging female employees to undergo sterilization, such a policy can certainly function as a powerful incentive to do so. If the company offers women alternative jobs, they typically pay far less, involve loss of seniority, and provide no opportunities for overtime. Many of the plants where such policies have been adopted are located in small one-factory towns; thus women who are prohibited from working in the factory may be unable to find work at remotely comparable wages—or any work at all. But the most telling flaw in the policy of protective discrimination is its failure to protect, because of the harm mutagenic substances can do to the fetus through the male.

The proposal that pregnant and nursing women, or women trying to become pregnant, be transferred to safe jobs at no loss of pay or seniority is invalidated by the same reasoning—it does not sufficiently protect. It is also likely to prove unworkable even as a means of protecting the fetus from nonmutagenic injury: the embryo is most at risk during the early stage of pregnancy, when a woman often does not know she is pregnant. (Fully 39 percent of pregnancies in the United States are unanticipated.)

In terms of social equity and the broadest possible protection of health, then, the most desirable approach appears to be to clean up the workplace by means of federal standard setting and regulation.

After an extensive review of the Occupational Safety and Health Act from the point of view of cost-benefit analysis, Robert Stewart Smith of the Cornell School of Industrial and Labor Relations reached the same conclusion: "By a process of elimination, then, it appears that an occupational health program must rely on a standards approach, despite its defects."[34] Smith's admitted reluctance to conclude as he does that there is no alternative to standard setting in matters of health—with regard to occupational *safety,* by contrast, he advocates the elimination of standards in favor of a species of market mechanism—may be taken as a more convincing testimonial to the necessity of standards than the advocacy of more eager supporters.

Standard setting and regulation is also, however, by far the most complex approach, involving as it does the most variables. As we shall see, the combined effect of these variables and the very nature of toxic substances themselves effectively preclude the perfectibility of the process.

*Constraints on Scientific Investigation*

OSHA standards specifically designed to protect against teratogenic, fetocidal, mutagenic, or carcinogenic effects would require the generation of data on a substance-by-substance basis, based on animal or bacteriological experiments, possibly in addition to epidemiological investigation of previously exposed human populations. Both kinds of investigation are plagued by serious methodological shortcomings. Let us mention just a few by way of illustration.

Some substances—thalidomide, for one—are not toxic to common laboratory animals; thus animal experimentation cannot be counted on to disclose all risks. Nor is an animal's lifespan necessarily equivalent to a human being's: that is, the fact that a rat does not develop cancer within five years of exposure to substance x does not mean that a human being will not get cancer twenty-five years after exposure. Epidemiological investigation is only feasible for substances that have been in use for some time, and such factors as women's name changes at marriage and the typical lack of information about the mother's occupation on birth and death records can seriously hamper epidemiological studies. Both kinds of studies are expensive and slow to produce results. These problems pertain to known toxic substances; clearly the identification of previously unrecognized toxins and the evaluation of newly invented substances pose further complications.

But let us assume, for purposes of discussion, that sufficient data have been collected on the effects of toxin x. What will be the nature of these findings? They will not as a rule demonstrate direct cause-and-effect in the sense that every exposure above a certain level produces a predictable outcome while exposures below that level have no ill effects. Instead, the results will be in the nature of a dose-response curve, demonstrating the variations in probability of a given ill effect at a given dose. An individual's vulnerability to harm may be affected by a number of factors, including duration of exposure and genetic susceptibility. Thus, even with the best conceivable data on which to base exposure standards, no standard above zero exposure can guarantee freedom from risk. The degree of risk may barely exceed the general risk of living or it may be massive, but risk attends any exposure to an airborne toxic substance.

Thus pursuit of the regulatory approach appears on ethical grounds to require full disclosure to prospective employees of whatever is known, and acknowledgment of whatever is unknown, about the extent of risk. (Such disclosure does not, however, affect the exercise of legal rights; a person cannot waive his/her own future rights or those of descendants, including the right to sue for damages.)

*Imperfections of Federal Regulation*

Even if the scientific findings were conclusive and unambiguous, the standards based on them would be subject to a number of other influences and ambiguities. For example, the Environmental Protection Agency, which administers the Toxic Substances Control Act of 1976, is required by law to ban or restrict the use of any chemical presenting an "unreasonable risk" of harm to health or the environment. The unavoidable ambiguity of the term makes it subject to alternative interpretations—and raises by implication the question of what constitutes *reasonable* risk. Whether the risk of exposure to a given substance is defined as reasonable or unreasonable is likely to be influenced by considerations of social benefit, availability of a substitute, and degree of exposure necessary (or, to put it another way, degree of protection feasible—and definitions of feasibility vary a great deal).

A proposed OSHA standard must go through twenty-two steps within the Labor Department, not to mention public hearings; at nearly all these points it is subject to modification. And, as Smith points out, "standards are enormously difficult to adopt or change if they are so stringent as to be controversial."[35]

Thus the regulatory process is not immune to political pressure, bias, expediency, laxness, or any other failing, and regulatory "imperfections" can have dire consequences. However, imprecision unavoidably characterizes every step in the process, including scientific investigation, and there is no single ready explanation for instances in which protective regulation fails to protect fully.

In sum, federal standard setting appears to be the most equitable and effective approach to protecting the health of workers and their offspring. But the conclusion is inescapable that, however thorough the research and however stringent the regulation of workplace exposures, occupational toxins will continue to cause an unknown degree of harm which can be characterized as neither residual nor negligent but inherent.

## Workplace Reproductive Hazards as a Public Issue

Popular journalism treats workplace hazards in a case-by-case fashion; science approaches the subject on a substance-by-substance basis. Furthermore, the risk is not yet sufficiently widespread to have aroused much public attention. Thus there has been very little acknowledgment of the predictability and severity of harm and virtually no recognition of the connection between advanced industrialization and mass consumption on the one hand and workplace hazards on the other. Another factor militating against such recognition is the prevailing assumption that science and technology are perfectible. Such an outlook further burdens the victims of workplace hazards in that no recourse has been made available to them except the courts of law, which are slow, expensive, and tend to put the burden of proof on the victim.

If we acknowledge the chilling reality that, even with full disclosure and stringent regulation, an unknown amount of permanent and severe harm will occur to workers and their offspring as a result of exposure to toxins in the workplace, we must confront a series of difficult questions. How should such harm be compensated? Who should bear the burden of proof? of cost? Could a compensation process be designed in such a way as to transfer the matter into the public domain, where the attendant issues of social values could be thrashed out?

## Compensation as a Potential Corrective

Federal tax-financed compensation for workers and/or their offspring permanently harmed by substances encountered on the job merits thorough consideration.[36] The major elements in such a plan would be a standardized schedule of damages and a board to hear individual cases. Like workers' compensation, this mechanism would simultaneously insure the worker against the economic effects of damage incurred and exempt the employer from liability for damage. It must be emphasized that a plan of this sort can only operate in conjunction with a rigorous regulatory system that sets and enforces standards of exposure on the basis of the best available knowledge. In the absence of strict regulation, tax-financed compensation would allow employers to neglect safety at little financial risk to themselves.

Those who attribute most occupational harm to the negligence and profit-orientation of employers might oppose such a no-fault plan on the grounds that it lets the employer off the hook, transferring to the public costs that the employer ought properly to bear. However, laying the burden of cost on the employer has distinct disadvantages. First, it puts the burden of proof on the employee, who must resort to the courts for redress. The disincentives to pursuit of a lawsuit—delay, expense, confusion, the uncertainty of the outcome—discourage all but a few victims from doing so. If the employer is found not to be legally at fault—if, for example, federal standards were complied with but were too lax or if the hazard was unrecognized—the victim can easily receive no compensation whatever. What if, as is particularly commonplace among women, the employee has had several employers? If after such a woman retires one of her children develops a form of cancer demonstrably related to her occupation, which of her employers is at fault? What if an employer has gone out of business by the time an occupationally induced disease manifests itself?

Enacting legislation to spread the risk across all taxpayers would also put the issue of workplace hazards squarely in the public domain, allowing for public pressure to be brought to bear on employers, legislators, and regulatory agencies. Public attention would thus be focused on the relationships among patterns of consumption, social values, and health. A case in point is nuclear power, whose future in the United States is uncertain because of intensifying public opposition. Spreading the risk across the public would serve to implicate all taxpayers in what would otherwise remain merely private misfortunes and isolated grievances.

A plan of this sort would also serve to create a centralized pool of data relating exposures to outcomes, which would be of immeasurable benefit for epidemiological purposes.

This discussion may appear to have wandered from the issue of employment of fertile women, but the inseparability of women, men, and children with regard to genetic and public health hazards militates against a more categorical approach. In sum, the effectiveness of federal standard-setting and regulation, in conjunction with full disclosure of the risks to potential employees, might be promoted by a system of publicly financed compensation for whatever harm nevertheless occurs.

## Conclusion

Working women's interests are not special interests. They coincide, by and large, with those of working men—and those of nonworking women as well. Overlap between the two groups of women is such that they are no longer really distinguishable: the huge majority of American women alive today, including those who are not currently employed, will spend a significant portion of their adult lives in the labor force.

Generally speaking, the labor market allows women to fulfill their family responsibilities only at a high cost in income, benefits, security, opportunities for advancement, anxiety, and future well-being. Women are penalized by corporate practices that treat full-time, uninterrupted employment as the norm and variations from that pattern as deviant. With regard to health, the practice of providing health insurance, disability insurance, and pension plans only for full-time workers is particularly onerous.

Attitudes have changed about the capacity of pregnant women to work, and the recent federal legislation will protect some women from discrimination on grounds of pregnancy. The overwhelming pregnancy-related problem facing working women, however, is not any of the circumstances surrounding the pregnancy itself—which is, after all, limited in duration—but how and under what circumstances a woman with an infant or small child manages to return to work at all. Because this is a matter not of discrimination but of job design, legislation cannot address it effectively.

Provisions that would greatly enhance the quality of life for employed women are workplace daycare centers, flexible hours, paid child-care leave (for either parent), job-sharing, and paid leave to care for sick children. Portability of pensions is a matter of particular concern to women. Anecdotal evidence suggests that at least some of the increased cost of such measures would be recouped in longer job tenure, increased efficiency, fewer sickdays, and the like.

Differences in physical capacity between women and men are of minimal significance in the labor market. Relatively few jobs demand the sustained expenditure of strength, and self-selection appears to weed out those of both sexes who cannot perform such work.

With regard to workplace hazards to fertility, the presence of women has simply highlighted an issue that threatens men in equal measure—and children as well, through the exposure of either or both parents.

In sum, women and men differ not at all in their need for safe workplaces. What special needs women have as workers grow out of their special role as the bearers and, usually, primary caretakers of children—and, as a consequence, their necessarily more flexible patterns of employment.

## NOTES

1. Kathryn E. Walker, "Household Work: Can We Add It to the GNP?" *Journal of Home Economics* (October 1973).
2. Louise Kapp Howe, *Pink Collar Workers: Inside the World of Women's Work* (New York: Putnam, 1977): 8.
3. Jerolyn R. Lyle and Jane L. Ross, *Women in Industry: Employment Patterns of Women in Corporate America* (Lexington, Mass.: D.C. Heath, 1973): 3.
4. Quoted in James W. Singer, "Affirmative Action for Jobs: Is the Sears Suit on Target?" *National Journal* (March 10, 1979): 388.
5. *Wall Street Journal* (November 14, 1978): 1.
6. Mitchell Meyer, *Women and Employee Benefits* (New York: The Conference Board, 1978): 15.
7. Howe, *Pink Collar Workers*, p. 253.
8. Meyer, *Women and Employee Benefits*, p. 22.
9. Charles E. Lewis and Mary Ann Lewis, "The Potential Impact of Sexual Equality on Health," *New England Journal of Medicine* 297 (October 20, 1977): 865.
10. Abstract of Constance A. Nathanson, "Illness and the Feminine Role: A Theoretical Review," *Social Science and Medicine* 9 (February 1975): 57–62, in *Women and the Health System: Selected Annotated References* (Washington, D.C.: U.S. Department of Health, Education, and Welfare, n.d.): 9.
11. Barbara Ehrenreich, "Is Success Dangerous to Your Health?" *Ms.* (May 1979): 53–54.
12. Hans Selye, *The Stress of Life* (New York: McGraw-Hill, 1956): 3.
13. Rachelle Barcus Warren, "Stress, Primary Support Systems and Women's Employment Status," testimony before the City of New York Commission on Human Rights hearings on women in blue-collar, service, and clerical occupations, April 22, 1975.
14. Lewis and Lewis, "Sexual Equality and Health," p. 866.
15. Ibid.
16. Ibid., p. 868.
17. Ibid., p. 865.

18. P. E. Enterline, "Sick Absence for Men and Women by Marital Status," *Archives of Environmental Health* 8 (1964): 466–470. Quoted in ibid., p. 865.
19. *Boston Globe* (May 29, 1979): 32.
20. Meyer, *Women and Employee Benefits*, p. 19.
21. Ehrenreich, "Is Success Dangerous?" p. 54.
22. Ibid., p. 98.
23. Rosabeth Moss Kanter, *Men and Women of the Corporation* (New York: Basic Books, 1977): 161–162.
24. *Boston Globe* (May 29, 1979): 32.
25. American College of Obstetricians and Gynecologists, *Guidelines on Pregnancy and Work* (Washington, D.C.: U.S. Department of Health, Education, and Welfare, Public Health Service, Center for Disease Control, National Institute for Occupational Safety and Health, 1977): 12.
26. *New York Times* (February 14, 1979): C7.
27. *Wall Street Journal* (November 7, 1977): 1.
28. William D. Kuntz, "The Pregnant Woman in Industry," *American Industrial Hygiene Association Journal* (July 1976): 424.
29. Jeanne Mager Stellman, *Women's Work, Women's Health: Myths and Realities* (New York: Pantheon, 1977): 152–153.
30. *Wall Street Journal* (August 1977): 1.
31. American College of Obstetricians and Gynecologists, *Guidelines*, p. 3.
32. Stellman, *Women's Work, Women's Health*, p. 161.
33. Ibid., p. 173.
34. Robert Stewart Smith, *The Occupational Safety and Health Act: Its Goals and Its Achievements* (Washington, D.C.: American Enterprise Institute, 1976): 84.
35. Ibid., p. 75.
36. This section is based on a proposal by Dr. William J. Bicknell, Director of Special Health Programs, Boston University Health Policy Institute.

## Discussion

**Stanley P. deLisser:** Ann Lebowitz has written an excellent paper that draws a very clear picture of the narrow range of relatively secondary jobs that are available to women.

**Donna J. Morrison:** Another thing that is nicely described in the paper is that women are now becoming heads of households and primary breadwinners. The problem is that the majority of the jobs that are available to women still reflect the assumption that the woman's income is secondary, even when ability is not a question.

**Eleanor Tilson:** The Storeworkers' Union represents employees of some major department stores in New York—Bloomingdale's, Gimbels, etc. These are places where women are concentrated and work primarily in low-paying jobs. We took a look at these jobs and noted that where people were in the top 10-percent wage bracket—mostly commission jobs such as furniture sales, rug sales, major appliances—these were the very departments that were dominated by males. Over the past five or six years our union has begun to take an active role on this, and, through collective bargaining, has won a clause which insists that when there are openings in these departments women have a right to move into them. It did not come without a struggle, but it is there now and slowly but surely there is a different mix in these departments. This is in unionized stores. As I move around the country in other cities I look in stores that are not unionized. If you walk into a furniture department or rug department, you will see mostly men. And yet these jobs are no more physically stressful than those in other departments of the stores.

We're also beginning to look into the question of what it means for people to stand on their feet for hours and hours on end. On occasion we have raised grievances about the issue of blood clots and vascular problems. Why shouldn't women be allowed to sit beside their counters when there are no customers to be helped? That, on occasion, seems to meet with some difficulty. These are real concerns.

**Richard H. Egdahl:** The Storeworkers' Union Security Trust has such good data—your hypertension studies, second surgical opinion trials, and so on. You say you see a lot of varicose veins in your members, and it's my impression that most are in older women who have had to stand at work as you describe. You could probably get some research-oriented surgeons to do a study to contrast populations who have the opportunity to sit down and relieve the blood flow versus a comparable group that has had to stand a great deal.

**Tilson:** That's a great idea.

**Jean G. French:** Some clarification is needed of Ann Lebowitz's discussion of NIOSH's testing program. While it is true that present knowledge of occupational toxins is limited, there is accelerated research activity in this area. NIOSH is conducting both epidemiologic and toxicologic research on acute and chronic effects from exposure to physical and chemical agents in the workplace. This research effort includes study of interaction between chemical agents, between chemical and pharmaceutical agents, between smoking and chemical agents, and between nutritional deficiencies and occupational exposures. The Toxic Substances Control Act stipulates that all new chemicals should be tested for adverse health effects prior to introduction into commerce. Section 4E requires that chemicals currently in commerce which have not been adequately tested should be tested with particular attention to carcinogenicity, mutagenicity, teratogenicity, and neurotoxicity. A federal interagency testing committee has been set up to identify such chemicals; it sends a list of chemicals recommended for testing to the administrator of the Environmental Protection Agency every six months.

**Leon J. Warshaw:** To comment on Dr. Bicknell's idea of a federally financed compensation system as described at the end of Ann Lebowitz's paper, I would point out that we are in an era of expanding federal government protection against the consequences of illness. That is evident in national health insurance proposals as well as in OSHA and the other protective legislation. With all these developments, and with workers' compensation as well as private, non–workers' compensation coverages, resources will be available one way or another to handle the health consequences to the individual who is damaged. Even the need of surviving infants who require lifetime care because of developmental defects will be covered one way or another. What the proposed approach will *not* do is provide punitive damages for wrongful death, wrongful life, pain and suffering, and so on, which lawyers will very quickly bring into the picture as ways of rewarding those who are successful in claiming negligence.

**William J. Bicknell:** So you say it will be very difficult to establish a barrier that would prevent the injured employee from going after the company?

**Warshaw:** Yes.

**Nina G. Stillman:** Workers' compensation was originally intended to be a bar to any further action against the employer and to avoid the need to go into the issue of fault. There was instead to be a state fund established, and employees who were compensated through the fund would then be barred from suing the employer in court. But in a series of cases over the last few years, the concept has fallen by the wayside. Employees are going to go after the employer anyway and the proposed federal no-fault system probably would not work.

# PHYSICAL CONDITIONING, STRENGTH, AND STAMINA

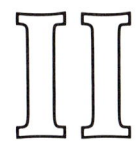

## II

# The State of the Art of Strength Testing

Joyce C. Hogan, Ph.D.

# 3

Employment selection procedures in settings that have historically employed a defined segment of the population are being scrutinized by both personnel administrators and industry applicants. The general level of knowledge, sensitivity, and action concerning equal employment selection procedures has increased significantly as employers make special efforts to hire persons, primarily minorities and women, who were previously excluded from full participation in the labor force. The principles of merit employment and fair employment are identical when merit decisions are valid: the goal is to establish personnel selection criteria that are neither arbitrary nor unrelated to actual job requirements. The importance of such criteria to potential employees cannot be overlooked: selection of employees who can perform the work required safely and successfully minimizes the chances of failure, low motivation, and job dissatisfaction, or subsequent dismissal. The employer, naturally, wishes to maximize the chances that employees will be able to perform the work effectively.

The involvement of women in jobs formerly performed only by men raises some critical questions where these jobs require either heavy manual work or prolonged exertion. It appears that a significant portion of women personnel may not be able to perform such work up to required standards, but some women can do so and some men cannot. Women should not, therefore, be denied these jobs on the basis of their sex. The problem is to establish the minimum standards that will assure effective job performance while allowing more women to qualify. This requires not only better methods of selection and training for physically demanding jobs, but also an analysis of physical performances actually required for certain jobs, and, in some cases, investigations of alternative job designs and performance procedures.

Some concepts and methodologies available from recent research can help to develop job-related, objective physical performance standards. This paper addresses considerations of preemployment selection procedures that involve muscular strength. Although physically demanding work may require other abilities as well,[1] strength is perhaps the center of physical performance variance. The discussion includes concepts and determinants of muscular strength, sex differences in base rates, assessments of strength requirements in work, and performance testing. The goal is to provide an understanding of the concept of muscular strength, especially as it relates to women, and its assessment in physically demanding work and in applicants for such work.

## Technical Considerations in Muscular Strength Testing

### Concepts and Determinants of Muscular Strength

Muscular strength is the ability to exert tension against an external resistance. Within this conceptualization, there are two factors that must be considered. First is the internal state of the muscle when under tension. If the muscle length does not change when tension is exerted, an isometric contraction results. If the muscle varies in length under contraction and the tension remains relatively constant, an isotonic muscular effort is the result. The second factor to consider in muscular strength is the accomplishment of mechanical work, defined as the product of weight and distance moved. In an isometric contraction the distance moved is zero, and no mechanical work is accomplished. However, since isotonic contractions change muscle length and affect joint action, mechanical work does result. The two possibilities of dynamic exertions occur, first, when the muscle shortens, and second, when it lengthens from a contracted position. Positive or concentric work is accomplished from muscle shortening; negative or eccentric work results from muscle lengthening. Astrand and Rodahl[2] contend that the mechanical model of work may be inappropriate for physiological considerations, and that work performed is relative to the product of developed force and contraction time. From this viewpoint, both isometric and isotonic contractions accomplish work.

Several factors account for both individual and group differences in strength performance. For purposes of selection procedure development, those factors concerning sex, age, and body size are of particular relevance, although some basic neuromuscular functions cannot be ignored. Maximal strength is proportional to the transverse area of the muscle: the larger the cross-sectional area, the greater the maximal strength. On the average, the maximal strength of identical muscle groups is greater for men than women. This is usually interpreted as a sex-linked genetic phenomenon that interacts with hormonal activity during ontological development.[3] Mean muscle strength across muscle areas of the body indicates that adult women's muscle strength is about two-thirds that of adult men. This is discussed in the next section.

Age determinants of strength have received considerable research attention, especially in children.[4,5] In adults, it is known that strength peaks between the ages of 20 and 30[6] and decreases progressively thereafter. Hettinger[7] reports that the maximal strength of a 65-year-old is 80 percent that of the original maximal. It appears that this decrement functions the same for men and women, with greater strength decline in the lower body extremities than in the upper extremities.

The ability people have to perform muscular work also has a mechanical relationship to the dimensions of the body and its extremities. The ratios between linear dimensions such as arms, legs, biceps, total standing height, etc., can be calculated for an individual, and, if one assumes geometric similarity across individuals, comparisons can be made and strength predicted. Based on these assumptions, Astrand and Rodahl[8] suggest that isometric strength varies with the individual's height squared. If there is geometric similarity across people, the taller person will theoretically be the stronger isometrically. Predictions of force or torque generated follow this same model of proportional linear dimensions, so that individuals with longer linear size can be expected to generate more force for performing work. Body mass or weight has an inverse relationship to both linear size (levers) and force (surface area). In this case, the larger, stronger person would be handicapped by the body weight in strenuous work performance.

Other physiological and mechanical variables that influence strength are of less practical significance for purposes of selection testing. Physiologically, muscle strength depends on the number of motor units activated and their tendency of contraction. Increases in external load require increases in motor units activated up to a ceiling at which the rate firing or contraction is responsible for further force increments. Fatigue, training, work recovery rate, available glycogen and phosphocreatine, and temperature can also affect individual strength. Mechanically, there is a point of maximal muscular tension, i.e., with the agonist slightly stretched that facilitates optimal muscular contraction. The strength of the contraction is diminished when the muscle is not on stretch, and the contraction cannot occur if the muscle is at its lowest length. For example, the optimum length of the biceps for muscle work is with an angle of 90 degrees at the elbow. Second, there are mechanical advantages associated with changes in joint angles. With an optimal angle, either extension or flexion will cause a decrease in the lever arm length and require an increase in muscle tension to balance the resistance. The third mechanical variable determining strength is cited by Morehouse and Miller.[9] They suggest that the arrangement of muscle fibers determine, in part, the force of the contraction with parallel fibers less effective than oblique fibers. That is, gains in power are caused by the increased number of muscle fibers occurring either in penniform (oblique) or bipenniform arrangement with the tendon.

## Sex Differences in Muscular Strength Base Rates

A literature review of strength research reveals that muscular strength interests not only exercise and work physiologists, but also industrial engineers, physicians, and psychologists. Research in industrial settings indicate manual work load capacities for women lower than those reported by work physiologists. Physiologists report the muscle strength generated by women as generally two-thirds that of men, but this generalization may not be particularly useful in light of differential upper and lower extremity sex differences in strength.[10] It appears that women's strength in the upper body extremities is considerably less than previously reported, but more than previously reported in the lower body extremities.[11,12,13] Laubach[14] reviewed nine research studies and found that averaging overall body strength masks the actual lever-relevant strength ratios between men and women. Four more specific muscular strength base rates derived from this review are upper extremity static strength, upper extremity dynamic strength, static trunk strength, and lower extremity static strength.

### Upper Extremity Strength

Women's upper extremity static strength ranges from 35 to 79 percent of men's with a mean of 55.8 percent. The following static strength measures were included in the analysis:

Forward push with both hands; reaction force provided by floor and footrest
Forward push with both hands; reaction force provided by vertical wall
Backward push with one hand; reaction force provided by vertical wall
Forward push with one hand; reaction force provided by vertical wall
Lateral push with the shoulder; reaction force provided by floor and footrest
Lateral push with one hand; reaction force provided by vertical wall
Vertical pull downward
Vertical push upward
Horizontal pull
Horizontal push
Neck flexion forward
Shoulder flexion
Elbow flexion
Elbow extension
Hand dorsal extension
Handle pronation
Handle supination
Key pronation
Key supination
Hand grip strength

At least three observations concerning these measures are worth note. First, vertical walls provide better resistance than floors (or horizontal surfaces) for arm-lever force generation. This may be due to the mechanical advantage gained in using strength from the leg position to augment arm force. Second, it appears that women demonstrate a higher percentage of strength in pulling measures than pushing measures. If this trend is valid, it follows that flexors in the arm levers can generate more static force than extensions. The third point is that data supported this prediction for both elbow and hand flexors, where flexors in both joints achieved a higher percentage of men's strength than extensors for those respective joints.

Measurements of upper extremity dynamic strength indicate that across the fourteen materials-handling tasks, women's dynamic strength ranges from 59 to 84 percent of men's with a mean of 68.6 percent (see table 1). These results support the static strength trends discussed above, with women demonstrating greater strength

## Table 1
### Measures of Dynamic Strength for Men and Women

| Measures | Median Values in Kilopounds Men's | Women's | Percent of Women's to Men's |
|---|---|---|---|
| LIFTING—Shoulder Height to Arm Reach | 22.2 | 13.2 | 50 |
| LIFTING—Knuckle Height to Shoulder Height | 24.1 | 15.4 | 64 |
| LIFTING—Floor level to Knuckle Height | 24.5 | 16.8 | 69 |
| LOWERING—Arm Reach to Shoulder Height | 20.0 | 13.6 | 68 |
| LOWERING—Shoulder Height to Knuckle Height | 25.0 | 15.9 | 64 |
| LOWERING—Knuckle Height to Floor Level | 28.1 | 17.3 | 62 |
| PUSHING | 36.3 | 27.7 | 76 |
| PULLING | 31.8 | 26.8 | 84 |
| STRAIGHT ARM CARRY—2.13 meters carry | 32.2 | 20.4 | 63 |
| STRAIGHT ARM CARRY—4.27 meters carry | 28.6 | 18.6 | 65 |
| STRAIGHT ARM CARRY—8.53 meters carry | 27.2 | 19.1 | 70 |
| BENT ARM CARRY—2.13 meters carry | 26.3 | 17.3 | 66 |
| BENT ARM CARRY—4.27 meters carry | 23.2 | 17.3 | 75 |
| BENT ARM CARRY—8.53 meters carry | 20.4 | 15.4 | 75 |

Sources: Adapted from S. H. Snook, C. H. Irvine, and S. F. Bass, "Maximum Weights and Work Loads Acceptable to Male Industrial Workers," *American Industrial Hygiene Association Journal* 31 (1970): 579–586; and S. H. Snook and V. M. Ciriello, "Maximum Weights and Work Loads Acceptable to Female Workers," *Journal of Occupational Medicine* 16 (1974): 527–534.

capacities relative to men in pulling tasks than in pushing tasks, and bent-arm carries (flexion) than in straight-arm carries (extension). It should be noted, however, that the absolute kilopound measurements are precisely in the opposite direction. Both men and women elicited more absolute strength in pushing than pulling and in straight-arm carries than bent-arm carries. However, the strength range for men across these tasks was nearly twice that for women, facilitating a greater percentage of women's to men's dynamic strength at the lower end of the measurement distribution.

*Trunk and Lower Extremity Static Strength*

Static trunk strength measurements for women ranged from 37 to 70 percent of men's with an average of 63.8 percent. The three tasks that provided these data were trunk flexion, trunk extension, and trunk bending sideways; different studies using these tasks showed considerable agreement.

Lower extremity static strength for women ranged from 57 to 86 percent of men's with a mean of 72 percent, based on measurements of:

hip abduction

hip adduction

hip flexion

hip extension

knee flexion

knee extension

ankle plantar flexion

ankle dorsi flexion

leg extension

These tests showed that sex-related strength discrepancies between the sexes are less with regard to the hip, knee, and ankle joints than any other body area.

*Relationships among Muscle Groups*

If these strength findings were averaged across the total body, women's strength would be about two-thirds that of men's. However, because of the magnitude of the differences between upper and lower extremity strength, an index of total body strength is meaningless, especially for predicting the ability to perform tasks involving specific levers or muscles. Measurements of the same nature as task content provide both content validity and job-relatedness. This view is supported by correlational analyses between muscle groups. Lambert,[15] using intrasubject comparisons, reports correlations of the same right and left muscle groups strength on the order of .80. Correlations between extensor and flexor strength in the same extremity were also high, but strength correlations for muscle groups across different parts of the body were rather low.

## Psychological Evaluations of Strength Performance

Perceptions of physical effort and difficulty interact with task performance at every level, but a comprehensive evaluation of their effects on physical performance has not been carried out. Two interesting studies that bear on this topic, Snook, Irvine, and Bass[16] and Snook and Ciriello[17] attempted to determine maximum weights and work rates psychologically acceptable to men and women. The studies were nearly identical in design and methodology, which permits comparison of their results. Work was manipulated in terms of independent height, weight, and rate variables with each of six manual materials-handling tasks for a total of fifty-four tasks. Subjects performing these tasks were instructed to adjust work load (weight) to the maximum amount they could perform without physical strain or undue exertion. Subjects had no information about the quantities of work they were performing; they were told to work at their psychophysical limit. This methodology is reviewed in detail by Snook.[18]

Results of the maximal acceptance weights and work loads in performing the 54 tasks were presented for industrial men (N = 28), industrial women (N = 15), and housewives (N = 16). Across all tasks, the maximum acceptable weight chosen by housewives was significantly less than for the other two groups. That chosen by industrial women was significantly less than that of men except for three tasks involving pushing and pulling. With fifty-four tasks, it is possible that these differences are artifactual, especially if the statistical treatment of mean comparisons was repeated t-tests. Multiple mean comparisons would resolve the question, but the authors did not identify the statistical techniques used. Also, maximum work loads (ft. lbs./min.) performed by industrial women were significantly less than for men with a few exceptions involving mostly high carrying tasks. Generally, women exhibited less variation and a narrower performance range than men.

Base rate results for sexes across categories of tasks support data discussed previously.[19] Sex differences were greater at slow than at fast rates of work: industrial women performed at 70 percent the rate of men during slow cycles and at 85 percent the rate of men during fast cycles. In terms of sex differences in maximal force acceptable in pushing and pulling tasks, industrial women exhibited 85 percent of the force produced by men. Results for lifting, lowering, and carrying tasks were slightly lower, with women working at 65 percent of the force of men. Housewives showed the same trends for both work rates and force results but the percentages were 25 to 30 points lower than for industrial women. These results are consistent with the earlier findings of Chaffin[20] and Nordgren.[21]

It is clear that muscular strength and muscular endurance as they interact with perceptions of exertion are an important component of objective strength performance. This psychological factor explains why persons of the same physical capacities may perform in dissimilar ways. A reasonable method to evaluate strength capacities is in terms of the percentage of population that can be expected to perform a task without discomfort or fatigue. This would lower the risk of injury or illness.

*Assessments of Strength Requirements in Work*

Only a few methods currently exist for assessing physical job requirements, and they vary in objectivity, sophistication, functional utility, and inherent psychometric properties. Observations and interviews are usually insufficient because they lack objectivity, do not lend themselves to systematic or quantitative analysis, and can give an unrepresentative sampling of the relative involvements of the different physical demands. Although somewhat more systematic in its procedures and classifications, the critical incident technique[22] lacks comprehensive evaluation of task components.

The *Position Analysis Questionnaire* developed by McCormick and colleagues[23] evaluates a number of job-analysis considerations. A particular strength of this approach is the consideration of frequency and importance of task performance. This method also includes a physical analysis of the job (e.g., physical exertion and body position). However, its limiting factor is that these categories are not sufficiently descriptive for analyzing strength and stamina requirements. Further, there is a considerable amount of overlap among the items, which leads to difficulty in identifying and separating the strength and stamina requirements.

Fine and Wiley's *Functional Job Analysis*[24] considers the stamina component of jobs but includes no strength factor per se. The strength component exists in several overlapping categories such as crouching, crawling, kneeling, and stooping. A further problem of analyzing more than one job or task is that the job requirement is evaluated as either present or absent. There is no evaluation of the amount of the capacity required, with the result that intertask comparisons are relatively imprecise.

Another source of job/task analysis, Comprehensive Occupational Data Computer Program (CODAP), is based on the results of Air Force job inventories. This approach uses numerous job/task statements taken from available job literature and supplemented by supervisors and technical school instructors. The inventory is administered to a large number of incumbents who rate each task they perform on a number of possible scales such as "relative time spent" and "amount of training needed." An important scale dimension concerns the index of "job difficulty." The definition of job/task difficulty finally selected concerns the "amount of time it takes for individuals to learn to perform the task adequately."[25] However, the concept of difficulty does not relate to the concept of physical demand in any systematic or categorical way.

*Physical Abilities Analysis* is an attempt developed by Fleishman[26,27] to translate the characteristics of jobs into physical requirements for personnel. This approach assumes that neither a general physical proficiency factor nor a general strength factor exists in performing physical work.[28,29,30,31] This result was obtained when actual performances were observed on several hundred physical proficiency tasks. People who performed well on certain groups of tasks did not necessarily perform well on others. The analysis resulted in nine factors that could account for the variance in physical proficiency of task performance.

The nine basic physical abilities that were found useful in describing hundreds of separate physical performances have been used to evaluate the physical abilities required in jobs and as a basis for selecting measures most diagnostic of the separate abilities. Four of the nine are strength factors.

The first of these is termed dynamic strength, defined as the ability to exert muscular force repeatedly or continuously over time. It represents muscular endurance and resistance to fatigue. The second factor, trunk strength, is a more limited dynamic strength factor—specific to the trunk muscles and particularly the abdominal muscles.

A third strength factor is static strength. In contrast to dynamic strength, which involves supporting the body's own weight, static strength is the force exerted against external objects (such as in lifting weights or pulling equipment). It seems to represent the maximum force that an individual can exert for a brief period; resistance to fatigue is not involved. The fourth strength factor is explosive strength—the ability to expend a maximum of energy in one or more bursts of effort, rather than in continuous exertion. Jumping tasks, for example, require this ability, as do short runs, but not longer endurance runs.

These strength categories are somewhat different in definition from those discussed earlier. This is probably because the former terms were developed by physiologists studying individual muscular functions, while the latter were defined by psychologists focusing on similarities in task characteristics. Fortunately, there is considerable overlap between the groups.

The Physical Abilities Analysis technique assesses the extent to which a job requires these four abilities plus the five that resulted from the original research. The technique has, for each of the nine abilities, a definition and a chart that differentiates it from the others. Accompanying each definition is a rating scale that includes concrete examples of tasks representing different amounts of that ability. For example, for "static strength," the 7-point scale goes from "requires little force to move a light object" to "requires use of all the force possible to lift, push, or pull a very heavy object." The specific task examples given range from "lift a package of bonded paper" (level 1 on the scale) to "lift bags of cement into a truck" (level 6). All scale values for task examples were determined empirically from previous research. In observing a new task, the rater looks at the activity involved with respect to the definitions and examples given and places it somewhere on the appropriate scale.

This method for assessing strength requirements in task performance has several advantages. First, a taxonomy-based approach provides a comprehensive assessment of all relevant physical strength factors within the defined physical domain. The analysis is both conceptually and theoretically complete. The major analytic problem for the field of job analysis is in translating the requirements of tasks to the capabilities of applicants. The Physical Abilities Analysis minimizes the inferences necessary for application because the terminology and concepts used are based on the abilities of people to perform tasks. Therefore, the second advantage is that the characteristics form a rather stable set of dimensions, while tasks are constantly subject to redesign. This approach is appropriate regardless of the task(s) evaluated. Finally, the method is practical, quantitative, and useful in large-scale administration across many tasks with physical demands. Much research has been conducted using the methodology and developmental efforts continue.[32]

*An Index of Perceived Physical Effort*

The idea that measures of perceived effort could serve as a basis for assessing physical requirements of jobs is virtually unexplored. This is surprising in light of the number of disciplines concerned with both work performance and effort.[33,34,35] Drawing upon several fields, some have tried to link empirically perceptions of physical effort with physiological work demands by means of a psychophysical assessment index.[36,37] It is necessary to demonstrate that individuals can estimate reliably the amount of physical effort necessary in task performance and that these ratings have validity for predicting actual physiological and performance costs of performing those tasks. This research has proceeded in two phases which investigate the psychometric properties and applied utility of a physical effort index in assessing real world task demands.

In the first phase, two investigations examined the relationship between ratings of perceived physical effort and associated metabolic expenditure. Tasks were rated on required effort by subjects who did not know the metabolic performance costs found in the physical work assessment literature. The first study found that personnel specialists' (N = 26) ratings of required effort were highly correlated with the known metabolic costs. The second study replicated the first using untrained male (N = 26) and female (N = 28) observers. No significant sex differences in rating were found. The two studies suggest a high level of agreement among subjects concerning the amount of effort they perceive necessary to perform a wide range of tasks. This was found for personnel specialists and for "untrained" subjects, both men and women. Also, the ratings of effort and the actual metabolic costs for tasks were highly related. The correlation obtained for one group of tasks was confirmed by a nearly identical correlation for a second group, both for personnel specialists and for a comparison sample. Thus, the data indicate high reliability and validity of perceived effort ratings over several types of task performances for both trained and untrained raters. Whatever sex differences existed in perceptions of effort for particular tasks are small or nonsignificant across a wide range of tasks. These results demonstrate that a perceived effort index can be used to assess the physical requirements of job tasks.

All the above ratings of task effort were made by subjects who did not actually perform the tasks. The second phase involved assessing the validity of the physical effort scale with actual task performance.[38] Twenty male subjects with no history of back or lower extremity muscular injury performed twenty-four standardized tasks in randomized order and rated them on a 7-point bipolar scale. Rating reliability assessed through intraclass correlation indicated substantial rater agreement, with a coefficient of .83. The major validity concern, the relationship between ratings of physical effort and actual work costs measured in foot-pounds, resulted in a correlation of .77, a substantial validation. Of specific interest for the present topic is the significant ($r$ = .86) relationship between physical effort ratings and weight manipulated in the tasks studied. Based on these results, regression equations were developed to predict both physical work costs and weight handled in materials-handling tasks from ratings of perceived physical effort.

The focus of this research was deliberately narrow. Because its focus is restricted to the physical domain, it provides more specific task information about physical demands more than global methodologies attempting to describe task requirements across a range of cognitive and psychological factors, but, on the other hand, its applicability is limited to the physical. The assessments of job requirements are rarely concerned about the psychometric validity of results, even though this demonstration is absolutely fundamental to any assessment device. The strength of the physical effort index is that ratings of physical effort are valid predictors of objective work requirements. Scale validation of this nature is a decided advance in assessing physical performance costs of work.

## Legal and Scientific Considerations in Muscular Strength Testing

The Uniform Guidelines on Employee Selection Procedures (1978) require the establishment of a valid relationship between a test or other selection device and actual performance on the job. Research strategies used to document the relationship fall into the categories criterion-related validation, content validation, and construct validation. From a legal perspective, it is ordinarily not necessary to validate selection procedures where no employment opportunities are denied on the basis of race, sex, or ethnic group.

Employers whose job classifications include heavy and very heavy physical work with emphasis on strength requirements are, no doubt, using selection practices with adverse impact for reasons of business necessity. Given sex differences in various strength capacities discussed earlier, selection procedures for heavy physical work involving strength will most probably result in adverse impact with regard to women and will require justification in accordance with the Uniform Guidelines. To date, a few employers have undertaken studies to demonstrate the relationship between tests and job performance, using either criterion-related strategies or content strategies.

### Criterion-Related Validity

Criterion-related validity refers to an empirical demonstration of a significant relationship between selection procedures and indices of job performance. Use of this strategy involves reviewing information about job requirements, determining important criterion measures, and choosing a pertinent trial test battery. Representative samples of subjects are tested in the trial test battery, placed on the job, and documented in terms of their performance on selected job criteria. The relationship between test scores and job criterion performance is computed and tests yielding correlations significant at the .05 level are retained. The final battery is determined according to the amount of performance variance accounted for by the component tests. These data are entered into a regression analysis, the result of which is an equation used for employment decisions.

The process of job analysis should lead to specification both of trial tests and of performance criteria. The two types of analysis most commonly used to evaluate the strength requirements of physically demanding work are biomechanical approaches and physical ability analyses. The former examine the content of the physical actions, express these actions in the content of tests, and devise or adopt a scoring system appropriate for the procedures. Work involving strength in any of eleven muscle groups can be assessed with well-known tests and measures (table 2).

Test development based on this approach is receiving large-scale validation in some armed forces divisions.[39] Specific biomechanical lever positions in relation to the testing apparatus were specified to reflect actual task mechanics for a wide range of tasks using various muscle groups. Three isometric tests assessed upper body strength, leg strength, and trunk extension of both male (N = 948) and female (N = 496) recruits. The resulting sample distributions of men's and women's scores indicate that females' upper extremity static strength was 56.5 percent of males', lower extremity static strength 64.2 percent, and trunk strength 66.0 percent. The lower extremity strength percentage is considerably lower than that reported by Laubach.[40] These tests will be used as part of a trial test battery and validated against performance on common soldiering tasks to predict successful physical performance during basic and job specialty training.

Chaffin, Herrin, and Keyserling[41] designed Standard Posture Tests that biomechanically simulated variations in lifting loads. These strength tests included simulations of lifting a compact object close to the floor using a leg/squat-lift technique, lifting a bulkier object from the floor using a back-lift technique, and lifting an object from a table or bench using an arm lift. Although this research was conducted to validate tests predictive of back injuries, the task simulation and biomechanical components of test construction are suitable for selection procedure validation.

A second type of job analysis, Physical Ability Analysis,[42,43] is a generic analysis attempting to categorize tasks according to descriptions of task strength dimensions derived factor analytically from over a hundred physical tests. Once a strength ability is identified as required for task performance, factor analysis review of the individual tests loading on the specific strength factor will provide tests most predictive of that strength dimension. Table 3 presents the four strength factors identified by Fleishman, the tests most predictive of each factor, test reliability, and primary factor loading. All tests are reviewed in detail by Fleishman.[44] Extensive normative data are available for these tests[45] but they are limited to male samples only. The male/female performance distributions on these tests is unknown in most cases.

Two recent criterion-related validity studies used the Physical Ability Analysis model as a basis for test selection. To implement physical

## Table 2
## Strength Tests for Defined Muscle Groups

| Reference | Grip/ Arm Static Strength | Arm/ Shoulder Dynamic Flexion | Arm/ Shoulder Dynamic Extension | Arm/ Shoulder Explosive Extension | Arm/ Shoulder Static Strength | Leg/ Hip Dynamic Extension | Leg/ Hip Explosive Extension | Leg/ Hip Dynamic Flexion | Leg/ Hip Static Strength | Trunk Dynamic Flexion | Trunk Dynamic Extension |
|---|---|---|---|---|---|---|---|---|---|---|---|
| Bookwalter (1943) |  | x |  |  |  |  |  |  |  |  |  |
| Clarke (1950) |  |  |  |  |  |  |  |  |  |  |  |
| Clarke (1966) |  |  |  |  | x |  |  |  | x |  |  |
| Clarke (1967) |  |  |  |  |  |  |  |  | x |  |  |
| Clarke, Bailey, and Shay (1952) |  |  |  |  |  |  |  |  |  |  | x |
| Clarke and Clarke (1963) |  |  |  |  | x |  |  |  | x |  |  |
| Cureton (1947) |  |  |  |  |  |  |  |  | x |  | x |
| Fleishman (1964) | x |  |  |  |  | x |  |  |  |  |  |
| Hunsicker and Reiff (1976) |  | x | x | x | x |  |  |  |  | x |  |
| Johnson and Nelson (1969) |  |  | x | x |  |  |  | x |  | x |  |
| Larson (1940) |  | x | x |  |  |  | x |  |  |  |  |
| Larson (1974) |  |  | x |  |  |  | x |  |  |  |  |
| Mathews (1973) |  | x | x |  |  |  |  |  |  |  |  |
| McHone, Tompkin, and Davis (1952) |  |  |  | x | x |  |  |  |  |  |  |
| Montoye and Lamphiear (1977) | x |  |  |  |  |  |  |  |  |  |  |
| Sharkey and Jakkula (1977) |  |  |  |  |  |  |  |  |  |  | x |

Sources:

K. W. Bookwalter, "Test Manual for Indiana University Motor Fitness Indices for High School and College Men," *Research Quarterly* 14 (December 1943).

H. H. Clarke, "Improvement of Objective Strength Tests of Muscle Groups by Cable-Tension Methods," *Research Quarterly* 21 (1950): 399–419.

H. H. Clarke, *Muscular Strength and Endurance in Men* (Englewood Cliffs, N.J.: Prentice-Hall, 1966).

H. H. Clarke, *Application of Measurement to Health and Physical Education* (Englewood Cliffs, N.J.: Prentice-Hall, 1967).

H. H. Clarke, T. L. Bailey, and C. T. Shay, "New Objective Strength Test of Muscle Groups by Cable-Tension Methods," *Research Quarterly* 23 (1952): 136–148.

H. H. Clarke and D. H. Clarke, *Developmental and Adapted Physical Education* (Englewood Cliffs, N.J.: Prentice-Hall, 1963).

T. K. Cureton, *Physical Fitness Appraisal and Guidance* (St. Louis: Mosby, 1947).

E. A. Fleishman, *The Structure and Measurement of Physical Fitness* (Englewood Cliffs, N.J.: Prentice-Hall, 1964).

P. Hunsicker and G. G. Reiff, *AAHPER Youth Fitness Manual*, rev. ed. (Washington, D.C.: American Alliance for Health, Physical Education and Recreation, 1976).

B. L. Johnson and J. K. Nelson, *Practical Measurements for Evaluation in Physical Education* (Minneapolis: Burgess, 1969).

L. A. Larson, "A Factor and Validity Analysis of Strength Variables and Tests with a Test Combination of Chinning, Dipping, and Vertical Jump," *Research Quarterly* 11 (1940): 82–96.

L. A. Larson, ed., *Fitness, Health, and Work Capacity: International Standards for Assessment* (New York: Macmillan, 1974).

D. K. Mathews, *Measurement in Physical Education* (Philadelphia: Saunders, 1973).

V. L. McHone, G. W. Tompkin, and J. S. Davis, "Short Batteries of Tests Measuring Physical Efficiency for High School Boys," *Research Quarterly* 23 (1952): 82–94.

H. J. Montoye and D. E. Lamphiear, "Grip and Arm Strength in Males and Females," *Research Quarterly* 48 (1977): 109–120.

B. J. Sharkey and A. H. Jakkula, *Development and Evaluation of Muscular Fitness Tests for Wildland Firefighters*, Special Report to Interagency Ad Hoc Committee on Muscular Fitness Testing, U.S.D.A. Forest Service Equipment Development Center, Missoula, Mont., February 1977.

## Table 3
### Physical Tests Predicting Strength Factors

| Strength Factor | Test | Reliability | Primary Factor Loading |
|---|---|---|---|
| Static Strength | Hand Grip | .91 | .72 |
| Dynamic Strength | Pull-Ups | .93 | .81 |
| Explosive Strength | Shuttle Run | .85 | .77 |
|  | Softball Throw | .93 | .66 |
| Trunk Strength | Leg Lifts | .89 | .47 |

Source: Adapted from E. A. Heishman, *The Structure and Measurement of Physical Fitness* (Englewood Cliffs, N.J.: Prentice-Hall, 1964).

selection tests for entry into outside craft positions, American Telephone & Telegraph used Physical Ability Analysis to determine the physical requirements of telephone climbing.[46] Factors of static strength, trunk strength, gross body strength, stamina, extent flexibility, and reaction time were rated required and critical to job performance. Tests predictive of each required ability component were entered into the trial test battery, administered to subjects (N = 210) entering pole-climbing school, and validated against time required to complete successfully a self-paced pole-climbing course.[47] Of the three tests retained for the final test battery, one was a measure of static strength. (See chapter 4 by Reilly.)

A second study involved devising selection procedures for entry-level order selector in a wholesale grocery warehouse. The job involved continual manual handling of grocery cases for 8-hour shifts, with the total weight moved typically exceeding 31,000 pounds per shift. The Physical Abilities Analysis revealed significant requirements for static strength, dynamic strength, and trunk strength. Strength tests selected for the trial battery included dominant and nondominant grip strength (static strength), push-ups (dynamic strength), and leg lifts (trunk strength). All entering employees were tested, placed on the job, and monitored in terms of objective production indices during a 30-calendar-day probationary period. Trial test battery means, standard deviations, and t-tests for men and women are presented in Table 4. Statistical analysis indicated that static and dynamic strength test results were significant and valid predictors of production indices.

### Content Validity

Selection procedures supported by content validity must be representative samples of the content of the job. The strength of content validity rests on the degree to which the selection content approxi-

### Table 4
Trial Test Battery Means, Standard Deviations, and t-Tests for Men and Women

| Test | Total $\bar{X}$ | S.D. | Men (N = 108) $\bar{X}$ | S.D. | Women (N = 21) $\bar{X}$ | S.D. | t(127) |
|---|---|---|---|---|---|---|---|
| Leg Lifts | 12.57 | (2.24) | 12.97 | (2.07) | 10.48 | (1.94) | 5.11* |
| Grip— |  |  |  |  |  |  |  |
| Dominant | 108.03 | (24.54) | 115.54 | (18.35) | 69.40 | (13.48) | 11.23* |
| Drip— |  |  |  |  |  |  |  |
| Non-Dominant | 101.37 | (23.38) | 108.32 | (17.71) | 65.62 | (14.75) | 10.36* |
| Push-Ups | 12.56 | (5.39) | 14.22 | (3.92) | 4.00 | (3.49) | 11.13* |

*$p < .001$

mates the content, complexity, and context of actual work behaviors. Job analysis results are typically translated into work sample tests which then assess applicant performance.

Two major limitations of content-valid physical strength tests concern the fundamental dependence on judgment in test selection and the frequent lack of scores from test administration. The nature of job content evaluation is subjective, although job content can be specified or evaluated using several different sources (e.g., subject matter experts, supervisor/incumbent ratings, etc.). The content domain is, in some sense, in the eye of the rater. Content agreement can be assessed across individuals and groups, but this reliability estimate does not impact the more important question of validity—that is, is the content selection a valid representation of the job? Schwartz[48] argues that every validation strategy requires subjectivity at some level, whether it occurs in the choice of a predictor test battery in the criterion-related strategy or the identification of traits to be measured in the content strategy. It appears that the more important issue is not whether subjectivity enters the process of validating selection procedures, but to what degree. On this point, it is clear that content validity requires significantly more human judgment than the other strategies.

Unfortunately, legal pressures and time constraints have encouraged employers to develop selection procedures quickly, and in some cases they are inadequate. Physical tests have been based on incumbents' false positive evaluations of tasks, infrequently performed tasks, hypothetical tasks, and tasks representing a statistically insignificant part of the job. Work samples requiring such actions as scaling a 6-foot wall or dragging a 200-pound dummy a specified distance should be carefully examined for valid test content.

The second limitation of some content-valid work samples is that they use only a discrete measure of pass/fail, precluding the range of scores that might be used for empirical validation. Since no variance is provided in work sample performance, no predictions can be made about on-the-job performance. A content-valid test is therefore meaningless in the classic psychometric sense.

In light of these shortcomings, it may not be productive to review content-valid strength tests in use today. Tests such as carrying a length of fire hose, ascending steps with emergency oxygen pacs, and rescuing a drowning "victim" reveal little about the future performance of a job. However, physical test development attempting to override these limitations can capitalize on the inherent strengths of the content-validity approach while avoiding the pitfalls. More innovative and relevant work samples are under development in the content-testing domain, although only a few exist for physically demanding work and many of these are limited to specific contexts.

A content-valid selection test for entry-level warehouse personnel was developed as part of the predictor battery in a criterion-related validation study.[49] The job required moving cases of products by hand from racks to pallets, and the primary indicator chosen for performance success was the number of cases moved per unit of time. With standardized work output, it was possible to specify case content representing 95 percent of the warehouse volume moved on the job. Further, given six storage locations in the warehouse, test cases could be located to represent a significant amount of case volume from each location. The relationship among volume outputs by location was also determined.

Work sample content was based on volume statistics indicating location of cases, representative case configuration for each location, and proportions of total cases moved from each location. Volume results were operationalized in a test whose physical features were a simulation of a warehouse situation. The test content, which required no training, was to select nineteen cases from predetermined locations and load them by hand onto pallets under speeded conditions. A continuous test score (total movement time for selecting and loading the cases) and a discrete score (cases omitted) were recorded.

Results indicated an immediate test-retest reliability of .77. The validity coefficient between the time required to complete the work sample test and a criterion (defined in terms of average number of cases moved per hour) was .36 ($p < .01$). The relationship between predictor tests based on physical ability constructs and work sample test scores were also significant and suggest factors underlying both work sample performance and measures of job success.

Although this work sample appears to have little generalization for use in other industrial settings, the model is prototypical. The basic requirement is that the job analysis take the form of a statistical frequency distribution which is then used to determine required behaviors. Any employer maintaining work orders, employee work distributions or plans, or production rates has the basic requisite for developing such a work sample. Next, the context in which the work is performed must be specified. From the output and the context, required behaviors are determined. Finally, the implicit or explicit criterion must be identified and quantified in terms of indices such as rates, time, or quantified ratings. The work context can then be simulated based on actual, not inferred, behaviors, scored, and validated against quantified criteria.

## Implications

Strength testing as a basis for personnel decisions requires more development and comprehensive conceptualization. We can no longer take tests measuring generic fitness levels and use them to predict success in specialized industrial settings. Job-related testing is now legally mandatory. Considerations of the applicants' abilities, review of job requirements, and objective assessments of both are essential. There are at least four issues implicit in the previous section that require discussion. The first two address problems of women and small-statured people in heavy work; the others concern needs of the testing enterprise.

Women, as a group, are at a distinct disadvantage in jobs requiring heavy, strenuous work. The data suggest that more women could perform successfully in some jobs than in others, but women as a group, will still be adversely impacted in hiring. The question employers will be forced to ask is whether job difficulty can be reduced through job redesign without undue expense in order to accommodate a larger segment of the applicant population.

Work procedures can sometimes be altered in the service of easing physical demands by clustering similar tasks or resequencing standard operating procedures. Fifty years of research from industrial engineering and time-study work has provided acceptable methods of redesign. For example, if a series of somewhat demanding tasks are performed successively, fatigue results, and fatigue tends to produce the perception of difficulty. However, if demanding tasks are sequenced such that easy or less demanding tasks are interpolated, fatigue can often be avoided.

Work aids can be developed to eliminate some of the demanding aspects of various tasks. In one example, the need to carry a heavy ladder from a truck to the job site was obviated by a specially designed wheel barrow (of nominal cost). The results of such work aids are often that many more women can perform the task and also that fewer men suffer back injuries.

A modification of work layout was completed in a warehouse operation.[50] This began with an analysis of the size and weight of cartons that had to be lowered, as well as the frequency of the need for them. The results indicated that many of the heaviest and most frequently needed items were located on 5-foot-high shelves. Furthermore, storage placement was typically independent of the size and weight. A simple redesign of placement permitted storage of 95 percent of all the warehouse volume on more easily accessible shelves.

A second area of concern to women entering physically demanding work is that some may be limited by inadequate physical capacity that job-related physical training could overcome. However, job-related remedial fitness programs are under way in surprisingly few industries, despite the benefits to be realized by both the applicant and the employer. Unfortunately, a change in this general policy will probably not occur until mandated legally.

A job-related training program for applicants entering physically demanding work is a no-lose proposition. First, the applicant has a higher probability of passing entry criteria for a job he or she wants. Second, the applicant is physically prepared for the work upon entry, reducing the possibility of injury and increasing immediate production. Third, the design of such a program is not a financial burden for the employer since it could be based on a job analysis completed previously. Also, these programs are usually self-administered off the employer's premises, thus eliminating the need to monitor or provide equipment for the program. Finally, the employer has a greater possibility of then finding women who can successfully perform the job. Such a program would probably not have an adverse impact on women, since available research suggests that there are no significant sex differences in the relative gains in strength as a result of training.[51] In light of the cost-benefit analysis, more employers whose jobs require heavy, strenuous work should consider implementing a job-related physical training program for applicants.

A third area of concern is the need for more objective, valid job assessment methodologies. This is a generic problem, not limited to assessments of physical requirements. As an assessment device, job analysis ought to be subject to the same psychometric requirements as any other assessment tool: that is, it should be standardized, objective, reliable, and valid. Further, information concerning these psychometric properties should be public, as it is for other assessment instruments. To become bona fide assessment tools, job analysis methods must relinquish the word of first-line supervisors as the sole unit of analysis, the dependence on a single "subject matter expert" for reliability, and the concept of rater consensus as validity. In physically demanding work, too many myths about job requirements are perpetuated by the self-interest of a few employees. This is not to say that employee interviews should be eliminated from job analysis, but rather that information from interviews should be only a part of a systematic procedure to gather job data.

The final concern is a need to develop more comprehensive and innovative physical tests. Tests validated using a criterion-related strategy usually have content validity as well as predictive validity, and they tend to be technically competent and defensible. Work sample tests for physically demanding jobs are usually insufficient for selection purposes. If content-valid selection tests are to become viable, they must overcome their traditional limitations with constructive, defensible alternatives. First, a content-valid selection strategy must have a system for scoring built into the device in order to fall within the definitional assumptions of traditional validity. Logically, if no scores result from the administration of a selection device, then there is no basis for inferences and predictions for employment success.

Second, more innovative methods for gathering job content data are necessary. Every widely accepted job analysis methodology is based on either ratings or judgments, but the validity of these methods for specifying job behaviors accurately is virtually unexplored. As long as job analysis depends on judgments, the content-validational strategy will be fundamentally subjective. Third, work sample selection tests should attempt to include as much job content as possible so that they realistically preview the job as a gestalt. To the degree this is accomplished, sole reliance on strength demonstration would be decreased simply because the strength requirements of tasks do not exist in isolation. Tasks typically require flexibility, speed, and coordination as well, and these factors often compensate for reduced strength.

## NOTES

1. E. A. Fleishman and J. C. Hogan, *A Taxonomic Method for Assessing the Physical Requirements of Jobs: The Physical Abilities Analysis Approach*, Technical Report (Washington, D.C.: Advanced Research Resources Organization, 1978).
2. P. O. Astrand and K. Rodahl, *Textbook of Work Physiology* (New York: McGraw-Hill, 1977).
3. E. Asmussen, "Growth in Muscular Strength and Power," in *Physical Activity, Human Growth and Development*, ed. G. L. Rarick (New York: Academic Press, 1973): 60.

4. H. H. Clarke, *Physical and Motor Tests in the Medford Boys' Growth Study* (Englewood Cliffs, N.J.: Prentice-Hall, 1971).
5. P. A. Hunsicker and G. Greey, "Studies in Human Strength," *Research Quarterly* 28 (1975): 109.
6. Astrand and Rodahl, *Textbook of Work Physiology*.
7. T. Hettinger, *Physiology of Strength* (Springfield, Ill.: Charles C Thomas, 1961).
8. Astrand and Rodahl, *Textbook of Work Physiology*: 123.
9. L. E. Morehouse and A. T. Miller, *Physiology of Exercise* (St. Louis: Mosby, 1967).
10. D. B. Chaffin, "Human Strength Capability and Low Back Pain," *Journal of Occupational Medicine* 16 (1974): 248–254.
11. E. Asmussen and K. Heeboll-Nielsen, "A Dimensional Analysis of Physical Performance and Growth in Boys," *Journal of Applied Physiology* 7 (1955): 593.
12. L. L. Laubach, "Comparative Muscular Strength of Men and Women: A Review of the Literature," *Aviation, Space, and Environmental Medicine* 47 (1976): 534–542.
13. B. Nordgren, "Anthropometric Measures and Muscle Strength in Young Women," *Scandinavian Journal of Rehabilitation Medicine* 4 (1972): 165–169.
14. Laubach, "Comparative Muscular Strength."
15. O. Lambert, "The Relationship between Maximum Isometric Strength and Minimum Concentric Strength at Different Speeds," *International Federation of Physical Education Bulletin* 35 (1965): 13.
16. S. H. Snook, C. H. Irvine, and S. F. Bass, "Maximum Weights and Workloads Acceptable to Male Industrial Workers," *American Industrial Hygiene Association Journal* 31 (1970): 579–586.
17. S. H. Snook and V. M. Ciriello, "Maximum Weights and Workload Acceptable to Female Workers," *Journal of Occupational Medicine* 16 (1974): 527–534.
18. S. H. Snook, "The Design of Manual Handling Tasks," *Ergonomics* 21 (1978).
19. Laubach, "Comparative Muscular Strength."
20. Chaffin, "Human Strength Capability."
21. Nordgren, "Anthropometric Measures."
22. J. C. Flanagan, "The Critical Incident Technique," *Psychological Bulletin* 51 (1954): 327–358.
23. E. J. McCormich, P. R. Jeanneret, and R. C. Mecham, *Position Analysis Questionnaire* (Purdue Research Foundation, 1969).
24. S. A. Fine and W. W. Wiley, *An Introduction to Functional Job Analysis: Methods for Manpower Analysis*, Monograph no. 4 (Kalamazoo, Mich.: Upjohn Institute, 1971).
25. R. E. Christal, *The United States Air Force Occupational Research Project*, Technical Report (Brooks Air Force Base, Tex.: Air Force Human Resources Laboratory, January 1974): 14.

26. E. A. Fleishman, *Physical Abilities Analysis Manual* (Silver Spring, Md.: Advanced Research Resources Organization, 1976).
27. E. A. Fleishman, "Evaluating Physical Abilities Required by Jobs," *Personnel Administrator* 24 (1979): 82–92.
28. E. A. Fleishman, *The Dimensions of Physical Fitness: The Nationwide Normative and Developmental Study of Basic Tests*, Office of Naval Research Contract Nonr 609 (32), Technical Report no. 4 (New Haven: Yale University, August 1962).
29. E. A. Fleishman, *The Structure and Measurement of Physical Fitness*. (Englewood Cliffs, N.J.: Prentice-Hall, 1964).
30. E. A. Fleishman, E. J. Kremer, and G. W. Shoup, *The Dimensions of Physical Fitness: A Factor Analysis of Strength Tests*, Office of Naval Research Contract Nonr 609(3), Technical Report no. 2 (New Haven: Yale University, August 1961).
31. E. A. Fleishman, P. Thomas, and P. Munroe, *The Dimensions of Physical Fitness: A Factor Analysis of Speed, Flexibility, Balance, and Coordination Tests*, Office of Naval Research Contract Nonr 609 (32), Technical Report no. 3 (New Haven: Yale University, September 1961).
32. Fleishman and Hogan, *Taxonomic Method*.
33. G. Borg, "Perceived Exertion as an Indicator of Somatic Stress," *Scandinavian Journal of Rehabilitation Medicine* 2 (1970): 92–98.
34. G. Borg, *A Ratio Scaling Method for Interindividual Comparisons*, Report no. 27, Institute of Applied Psychology (University of Stockholm, 1972).
35. G. Borg and B. J. Noble, "Perceived Exertion," in *Exercise and Sport Sciences Reviews* ed. J. H. Wilmore, vol. 2 (New York: Academic Press, 1974).
36. J. C. Hogan and E. A. Fleishman, "An Index of the Physical Effort Required in Human Task Performance," *Journal of Applied Psychology* 64 (1979): 197–204.
37. J. C. Hogan, G. D. Ogden, D. L. Gebhardt, and E. A. Fleishman, *Methods for Evaluating the Physical and Effort Requirements of Navy Tasks: Metabolic, Performance, and Physical Ability Correlates of Perceived Effort*, Technical Report (Washington, D.C.: Advanced Research Resources Organization, 1979).
38. Ibid.
39. J. Knapik, D. Kowal, P. Riley, J. Wright, and M. Sacco, *Development and Description of a Device for Static Strength Measurement in the Armed Forces Examination and Entrance Station*, Technical Report (Natick, Mass.: U.S. Army Research Institute of Environmental Medicine, 1979).
40. Laubach, "Comparative Muscular Strength."
41. D. B. Chaffin, G. D. Herrin, and W. M. Keyserling, "Preemployment Strength Testing," *Journal of Occupational Medicine* 20 (1978): 403–408.
42. Fleishman, "Evaluating Physical Abilities."
43. Fleishman and Hogan, *Taxonomic Method*.
44. Fleishman, *The Structure and Measurement*.
45. Ibid.

46. S. Zedeck, *Validation of Physical Abilities Tests for PT&T Craft Positions*, Technical Report no. 7 (Basking Ridge, N.J.: American Telephone & Telegraph, January 1975).
47. R. R. Reilly, "Physical Ability Test Measures Related to Performance in Physically Demanding Jobs," Paper presented at American Psychological Association Annual Meeting, Toronto, Canada, August 1978.
48. D. J. Schwartz, "Content Validation," Paper presented at IPMA Selection Specialists' Symposium, Chicago, July 1976.
49. J. C. Hogan and W. Barlow, "Toward Defensible Content Valid Work Samples," Working Paper (Washington, D.C.: Advanced Research Resources Organization, 1978).
50. J. C. Hogan, G. D. Ogden, and E. A. Fleishman, *Validation of a Physical Ability Test Battery for Entry-Level Warehousing Jobs*, Final Report (Washington, D.C.: Advanced Research Resources Organization, 1979).
51. J. H. Wilmore, "Alterations in Strength, Body Composition, and Anthropometric Measurements Consequent to a 10-Week Weight Training Program," *Medicine and Science in Sports* 6 (1974): 133–138.

# Moving Women into Outside Craft Jobs

*Richard R. Reilly, Ph.D.*

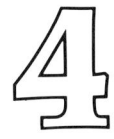

# 4

As part of a 1973 consent decree with the federal government, AT&T and the Bell System agreed to hire specific percentages of minorities and females into certain jobs. After the decree took effect, significant numbers of women were hired for the first time in outside craft jobs: cable splicing, line construction, and the installation and repair of outside plant. It was not too long before problems became apparent. The dropout rate for women in these jobs was over 50 percent within the first six months, with half the dropouts leaving during training. The rate of injury for women was extremely high, particularly of injuries occurring during pole climbing.

Almost all outside craft workers must at some time climb telephone poles in the course of their jobs. The Bell System has two kinds of poles. In the familiar "stepped" pole, metal protrusions or "steps" are permanently mounted and are used by the worker to climb. The other kind, the unstepped pole, must be climbed with a tool called a climber.

The standard Bell System climber, shown in figure 1, consists of a long shank shaped at its lower end into a stirrup. A sharp gaff is welded to the bottom of the shank, and its top is fitted with an adjustable extension sleeve that enables the user to fit the climber to his or her leg. The climber is strapped around the leg with the shank on the inside and the instep fitting over the stirrup. The employee climbs by jabbing the gaff into the pole. An accident on an unstepped pole usually occurs when the gaff cuts through and out of the pole. This is referred to as a cutout. At this point, the employee may fall backward off the pole or, if using a safety belt, slide down the pole. The risk of injury is great in either case.

## Problem Survey and Response

The injury rate for females climbing unstepped poles was extremely high—in some cases, nine times higher than the men's rate. This, plus the turnover rate and other problems reported by the field, led the Bell System to undertake a survey of women working in outside craft jobs. This survey, completed in 1976, sampled almost all women and a comparison group of men working in outside craft positions in four Bell System companies. Women reported many more problems in almost all areas. They were much more likely to be tired at the end of the day, either in training or on the job, and more likely to have problems related to strength factors and to the use of equipment. Most disturbingly, many more women fell while in pole-climbing training than did men, though a fall does not always lead to an injury.

It was clear from the survey and field reports that women were having a number of specific problems which should be addressed. In response, the Bell System instituted revisions in equipment and tool design, training methods, selection, and the design and organization of work.

One of the first steps taken was to review the availability of suitable equipment for women. Most of the available equipment—work gloves, boots, rain gear, safety belts, etc.—was designed for a relatively large male. Small females in particular had problems in using this equipment. Manufacturers were contacted and in most cases equipment suitable for smaller people was identified and made available. In some cases, however, suitably modified equipment did not exist. This was true, for example, of the climbing tool described earlier. A specific developmental effort was then undertaken to develop a new small climber for women.

The problems mentioned by women in the survey with training methods and procedures appeared to be consistent with reports from

Moving Women into Outside Craft Jobs 101

**Figure 1**
Standard Bell System F-Type Climber (A pad that fastens to the top of the shank is not shown here.)

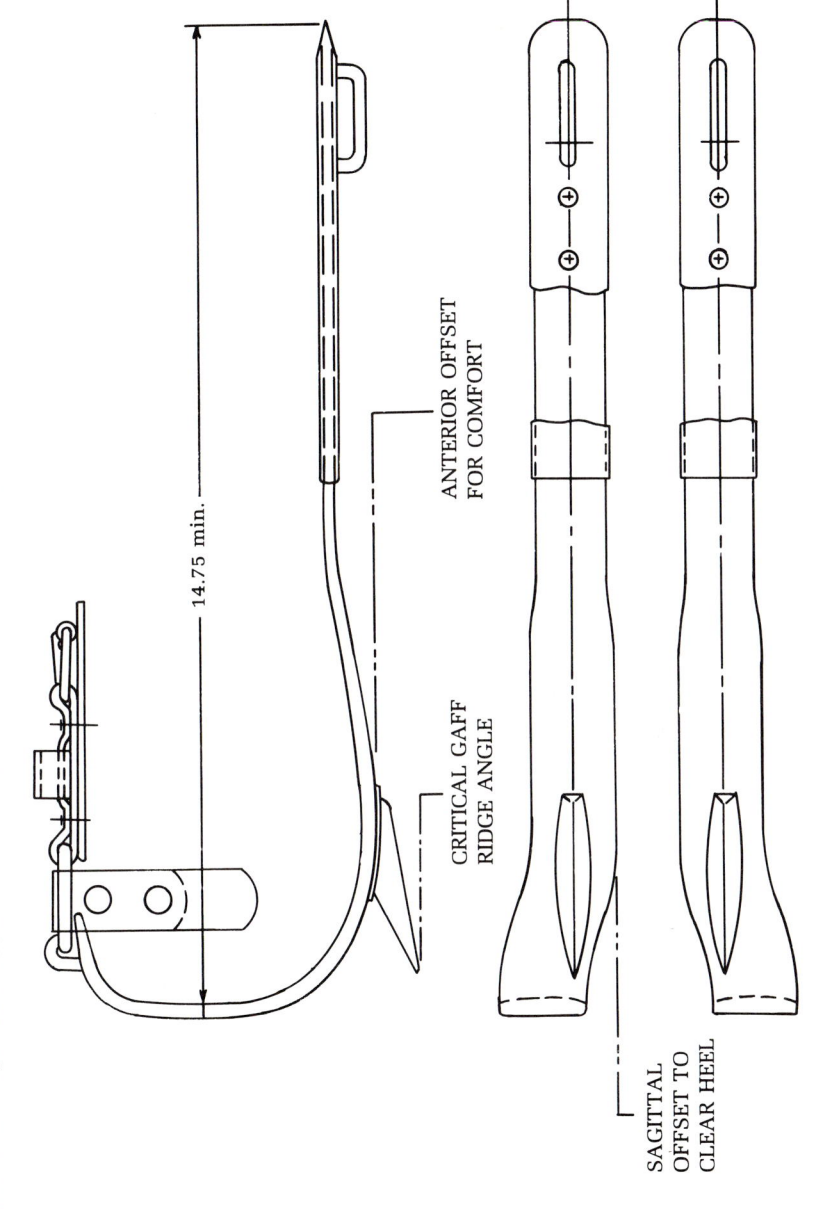

the field. Thus, a second effort was to revise the pole-climbing training and institute a new Bell System standard pole-climbing course.

A third area of concern was the physical status and conditioning of women (and men) who were going into outside craft work. Identifying a method of selecting persons with suitable physical abilities to undertake the pole-climbing tasks became a major effort.

Finally, a variety of alternative approaches to the task of pole climbing and to outside craft work were and are being considered. These include such possibilities as the reorganization of work in outside craft and the use of various aids and devices that would eliminate the need for climbing unstepped poles with climbing tools.

## Development of a New Small Climber

The original climbing tool design has been used for over seventy years with little evidence of problems. As women and other people of small stature began to come into pole-climbing jobs, however, it became apparent that the design was not suitable. The angle of the gaff on the climber is considered critical, since a less than optimum angle can create great strain on the pole climber and also increase the probability of a cutout on the pole. The standard climber has a gaff angle of 12 degrees. A biomechanical study which compared the male and female physiques with respect to the pole-climbing task suggested that a gaff angle of 15 degrees might be more suitable for women.[1]

In 1977 four different prototype small climbers were developed. One of these had the standard angle of 12 degrees, another had an angle of 18 degrees, and two others had 15-degree angles. One hundred female pole climbers from various Bell System locations participated in a trial designed and analyzed with the assistance of human factors specialists from Bell laboratories. All women had been trained in pole climbing and used climbers as part of their regular work assignment.

Wearing a harness to prevent falls, each of the subjects tested each of the trial climbers by ascending the pole to a working height, maneuvering to the right and left, maneuvering in a vertical plane, and descending the pole. Subjects made five climbs a day for two consecutive days, with suitable rest periods between climbs. An administrator observed each subject climbing and maneuvering on the pole with each of the prototype climbers to note any climbing deviations. After each climb, the subject completed a survey form evaluating the climber and commenting on such factors as leg comfort, penetration of gaff, and relative ease of climbing. Results clearly indicated that the new climber with the 12-degree angle was preferred. This new climber is now made available to all personnel as an option to the standard Bell System climber and is the tool most often used by females.

## Pole-Climbing Training

A major effort to revise Bell System Pole-Climbing Training began with a detailed analysis of the tasks involved in pole climbing. This led to the development of a specific series of training objectives for the new self-paced course. Training is now divided into six major parts. Ladder Handling covers the use and safe handling of extension ladders; Introduction to Pole Climbing introduces methods and general safety; Climbing Fundamentals covers fitting, wearing, maintaining, and using the body belt and safety strap; Beginning Climbing Skills includes the use of climbing gear on stepped and unstepped poles; Building Climbing Skills covers maneuvering, reaching, and working aloft; Avoiding Climbing Hazards covers preclimbing checks of poles and safety behavior while working aloft. These major parts are broken down into subunits, each with an attached mastery test which the trainee must pass before proceeding to the next. The entire course is self-paced and each trainee receives a great deal of individual attention. With such a course, most of the failure is self-motivated.

Several other features of the course are worth mentioning. First, trainees are video taped while climbing and then allowed to view their performance with an instructor who critiques the performance. This method of feedback has proven quite successful. Second, the pole climbing is done in half-day sessions to alleviate the problem of fatigue. During the rest of the day, trainees learn other (nonphysical) aspects of the job. Finally, all trainers are certified by a rigorous procedure which ensures that certain minimal standards for proficiency are met. All training facilities are monitored and trainers are evaluated regularly.

## Physical Ability Testing

It is certainly no surprise that males and females differ in physical abilities, particularly in gross physical strength. Problems reported from the field and from our survey indicated that we needed a selection procedure focused on the particular physical abilities needed to perform pole climbing. The first step was to analyze the pole-climbing job in terms of both the tasks and the abilities required. The analysis was greatly facilitated by a set of behaviorally anchored rating scales developed by Theologus, Romashko, and Fleishman, which cover a wide range of both physical and cognitive abilities.[2] Each scale is defined generally and its high and low ends are described. Specific examples of behavior then serve to anchor points on the scale. See figure 2 for an example. The scales have been used with success in a variety of contexts and are used extensively in our own job analysis work.

Supervisors and incumbents in several different locations in the Bell System provided data on the importance of various tasks and

**Figure 2**
Sample Physical Abilities Scale: Static Strength

This is the ability to use *continuous* muscle force to lift, push, pull, or carry objects. This ability can involve the hand, arm, back, shoulder, or leg.

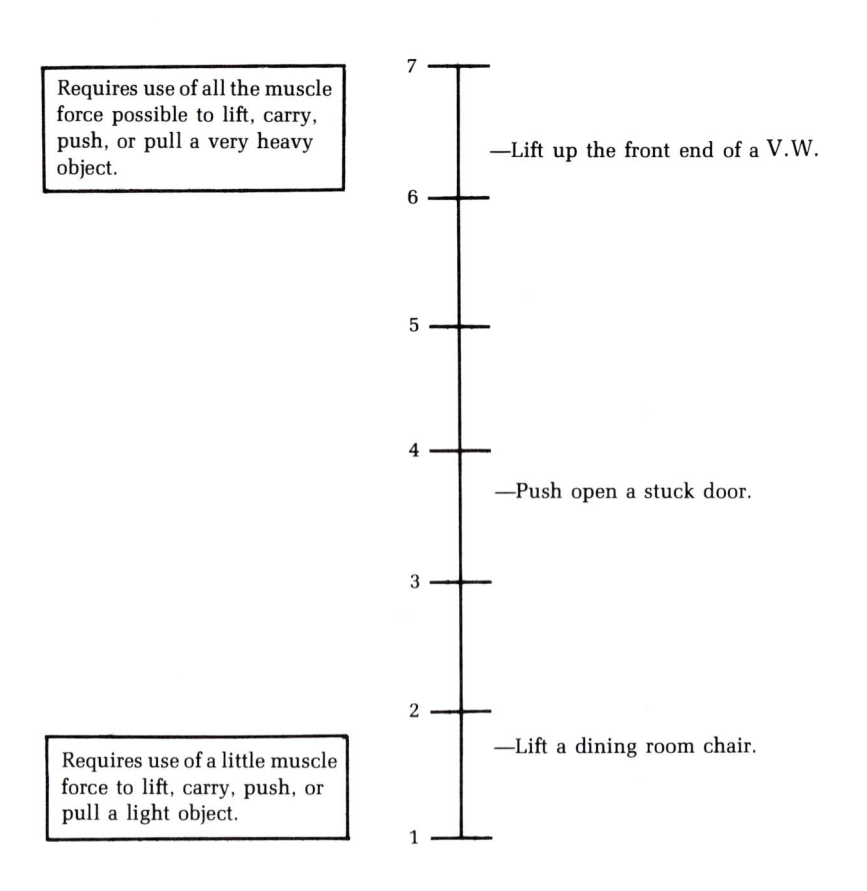

| | | |
|---|---|---|
| Requires use of all the muscle force possible to lift, carry, push, or pull a very heavy object. | 7 —<br>6 — | —Lift up the front end of a V.W. |
| | 5 — | |
| | 4 —<br>3 — | —Push open a stuck door. |
| Requires use of a little muscle force to lift, carry, push, or pull a light object. | 2 —<br>1 — | —Lift a dining room chair. |

abilities. Based on these data, plus interviews and observation, a battery of physical measures was recommended.

Grip strength: measured by taking the average of three trials with a hand dynamometer which recorded kilograms force

Dynamic trunk strength: measured by counting the number of sit-ups achieved in 30 seconds with a 10-pound weight behind the head

Reaction time: measured by taking the average number of milliseconds to respond appropriately to one of three possible visual stimuli (lights) over ten trials

Dynamic arm strength: measured by counting the number of revolutions achieved in 60 seconds while pedaling a bicycle ergometer with the hands (resistance on the ergometer was set at 3 kilograms)

Dynamic leg strength: measured in a similar way while pedaling the ergometer in a normal manner

Balance, or gross body equilibrium: measured by taking the total time that a subject could balance on one foot on a ¾-inch balance beam over two trials

Static arm and shoulder strength: measured by taking the average force achieved over three trials by pulling a cable across the chest (a tensiometer was used to record the force)

Stamina: measured with the Harvard Step Test, recording both the Harvard Step Index, a function of total time achieved in heart recovery rate, and the total time achieved in seconds

Extent flexibility: measured by the distance the subject's arm could be extended in a rotating stretch of the trunk

Body density: derived from measurements of the subcutaneous fat at specific body sites (for males, the front of the thigh and the subscapular area; for females, the suprailiac and triceps areas)

Other measures of resting heart rate, height, weight, arm span, and arm reach

All these tests and measurements were recorded for a sample of 210 job candidates (78 females and 132 males) representing six different Bell System locations throughout the country. Each subject was scheduled for pole-climbing training and had thus qualified with respect to paper-and-pencil tests and the usual company medical examination. Although subjects went through all the physical tests and measurements, data were reported neither to the subject nor to anyone in the field. All subjects went into pole-climbing training regardless of their test performance, and no decisions or actions were taken based on any of the data during the study.

We then followed each subject through training and into the job, taking performance measures at several different points. Because of the self-paced nature of training, training performance was measured by the time taken to complete the course. (A second measure was whether the trainee left or dropped out of training for physical reasons.) Pole-climbing proficiency on the job was evaluated at weekly intervals for four weeks, using a standard checklist. Each candidate had to perform a series of exercises in ascending, descending, and maneuvering on the pole. Finally, all accidents related to pole climbing were recorded for the trainees for a period of six months.

We now had two sets of scores or data: the physical ability measurements taken before training and the performance measures taken for training and work proficiency. A series of correlation computations then identified the best subset of predictors. For this we used a stepwise procedure which begins with the most predictive physical ability test and then adds to it each next-best predictor of later performance. To anyone familiar with this statistical procedure, it is no surprise that the increase in prediction drops off rather sharply after the first few variables have been added. The best predictors turned out to be the body density, static strength, and balance; a score based on these three tests was predictive of all our measures of training and job performance. Adding remaining tests did not significantly increase prediction.

The federal government's Uniform Guidelines on Employee Selection Procedures specify in great detail the documentation necessary to support a procedure that is likely to have adverse impact on a protected group.[3] In the case of the physical abilities test, there was little doubt that females would fail the test more often than males. It became important, then, to ensure that the test met the government's guidelines as well as those advocated by the profession of industrial psychology. The most important factor is whether the test is fair, in the sense that it predicts in the same way for each group. The analysis indicated that the test predicted in about the same way for females as for males; in fact, where there were differences, the test appeared to predict better for females.

We now had a test that met the definitions of fairness and appeared to be a valid, job-related predicator. It so happened that we had taken another sample for a preliminary study, forty-two females and eighty-six males, for whom we also had physical test data, training performance measures, and accident data. As a cross-check, we correlated our test battery scores with three indices of performance in this new sample and found that they significantly predicted training performance, turnover, and accidents. These results suggested that our battery should be implemented and used for selecting applicants for pole-climbing jobs. Table 1 summarizes the correlations we found in both samples.

### Table 1
Correlations between Final Physical Test Battery and Measures of Training and Job Performance

| Measure | Sample Size[a] | Correlation[b] |
|---|---|---|
| Training Performance | 177 | .46 |
| Training Dropout | 192 | −.38 |
| Field Review | 96 | .36 |
| Accidents | 318 | −.15 |
| Training Performance[c] | 142 | .31 |
| Dropout[c] | 142 | −.33 |

[a] Sample sizes varied because it was not possible to collect all data on all subjects.
[b] All correlations significantly different from zero with probability less than 0.01.
[c] Preliminary study.

In 1978 the test became a Bell System requirement of all applicants for an outside craft job that required pole climbing. By now we have tested thousands of applicants, and our results indicate that we can expect about half or more of the females to fail but only 10 percent or less of the males.

## Other Approaches

Several other approaches to pole climbing that do not require the climbing tool are under consideration. One such device is actually a portable ladder that fits around the pole and can be used without much risk of injury. A second device consists of a seat and a foot rest each with an attachment that encircles the pole. The employee ascends the pole by first standing on the footrest and lifting the seat and then sitting on the seat and lifting the footrest with the legs. The edges of the seat and footrest are set at an angle to the pole so that slipping is virtually impossible. Preliminary field trials indicate that people can use the device safely with very little training. These devices and others are being field tested and if one or more of them proves successful, the use of conventional climbers may diminish significantly.

Another trial, still being evaluated, examined ladders as an alternative to climbers. Ladders are not appropriate for some situations, but they may be a safer alternative for most climbs of unstepped poles. Finally, we are examining the possibility of reorganizing the outside craft job into climbing and nonclimbing specialties. There is some evidence that a fairly small number of specialists in pole climbing could handle most of the climbs necessary. This would reduce the total number of outside craft workers engaged in pole climbing, and also limit pole climbing to employees who climb on a regular basis, thereby maintaining their skills at a high level.

It is worth noting that although a reexamination of the pole climbing component of outside craft work was a direct result of the influx of women into these jobs, the changes that have resulted apply to all workers. Besides reducing the dropout and injury rates for females, the changes should also benefit the male craft work population.

---

**NOTES**

1. M. J. Brookes, *A Biomedical Study of the Problems Faced by Women When Climbing Poles with the Use of Leg-Mounted Climbing Irons* (New York: American Telephone and Telegraph Co., 1975).
2. G. C. Theologus, T. Romashko, and E. A. Fleishman, *Development of a Taxonomy of Human Performance: A Feasibility Study of Ability Dimensions for Classifying Human Tasks*, Tech. Rep. 726–5 (Washington, D.C.: American Institutes for Research, January 1970).
3. "Uniform Guidelines on Employee Selection Procedures," *Federal Register* (August 25, 1978): 38290–38315.

## Discussion

**Richard H. Egdahl:** When someone, say a male, enters an outside craft job, how long does he stay at it? Does he move on to other jobs, or is that a job he enters and stays in for the rest of his life?

**Reilly:** We have a variety of craft jobs, and workers can and often do stay in outside craft work with the pole-climbing requirement as part of the job for virtually an entire career.

**Jeanne M. Stellman:** Have you broken down your employees into age groups and studied accident and injury rates by age? In other words, how does the accident and injury rate of 50-year-old male pole climbers compare with 25-year-old male pole climbers and with females?

**Reilly:** No, we haven't looked at that. As you know it is difficult to do controlled studies of accidents. We did look at all accidents that occurred among people going through our pole-climbing training program, and even there we found a very large difference in the accident rate for women versus men.

**Egdahl:** How do people get assigned to these jobs?

**Reilly:** The normal procedure would be first a paper-and-pencil test to measure your ability to learn the other aspects of the job. Then only those going into pole-climbing jobs have to pass the physical test.

Those assigned to a downtown metropolitan area with no telephone poles would have no need for the physical abilities test for pole-climbing training. In some cases a worker might be sent to pole-climbing school after years on the job upon reassignment to a job requiring a lot of pole climbing.

**Eleanor Tilson:** Many women would not particularly consider pole climbing. Did the company do any testing on the manual dexterity capabilities of women as opposed to men? It seems to me the Bell System must have many jobs—very delicate wiring and that kind of thing—that women could perform well. Was such testing done at all?

**Reilly:** No. The Bell System has been adopting forms of technology which have made it much, much simpler to do the wiring and connecting needed to maintain a telephone system. If you look at the cable splicing done today, the manual requirements are far less than they were, say, ten years ago. There is, I think, enough general evidence available to support your point that women do have better manual dexterity. And in the future we may be moving toward another new technology where very fine filaments are used to carry telephone messages with light. This does require a great deal of visual and motor coordination, and it could be that women will actually be better at that than men. At this point, however, our workers just don't have a problem with the manual dexterity requirements of craft jobs.

**Leslie I. Boden:** It seems to me that we should take a broad look at this problem for a moment. Both men and women generally prefer good jobs to bad jobs. They avoid repetitive jobs with low pay and tight supervision, and prefer flexible jobs with high pay. Craft jobs in the Bell System seem to be good jobs, but jobs that, because of current physical requirements, are not available to many women. This leads me to two questions. First, within the Bell System now, how many craft jobs are there, and how many of them are inside, that is, available to women regardless of physical conditioning? Second, if Bell changed the organization of outside work to make pole climbers a smaller, specialized group, how many new outside jobs would be opened to women and men without the superior physical abilities required to climb poles safely?

**Reilly:** I can't give you exact numbers. We have 100,000 people in our outside craft jobs, and inside probably something like 80,000. The inside jobs are open to women and do not pose the same physical ability problems. One reason we're looking at the possibility of reorganizing the outside jobs so that we have a smaller number of specialists who do a lot of pole climbing on a regular basis is that the skills required for pole climbing are not maintained unless they're used regularly.

**Boden:** I'm struck by the amount of effort that has been devoted to trying to find good physical tests and by the attention that has been paid to the conditioning of female job applicants. It seems that the approach you have just suggested could produce preferable results for both worker safety and equal opportunity. If, out of 180,000 craft people there were 10,000 pole climbers instead of 100,000, then the issue of women getting good craft jobs in the Bell System would not hinge so heavily on their being able to climb poles safely. In addition, the more specialized pole climbers would climb poles more regularly than outside craft people do now, and would therefore be more skilled and safer. It strikes me that the majority of AT&T's effort might well be devoted to restructuring the occupational requirements of craft jobs, opening them to more people rather than trying to restructure the people to fit into current occupational requirements.

**Reilly:** That's one option we are exploring. Another is to develop ways to climb poles that don't require that much physical strength, as discussed in my paper. These are being tested now and could probably eliminate all but a very few instances where a pole would have to be climbed in a manner requiring a lot of physical capability. The option of restructuring the jobs is one that would be a substantial departure from past practice. It involves a lot of resistance, particularly in a large organization. And there's the counterargument, "Suppose we have an emergency, a hurricane for example, where we need large numbers of people to go out into the field and climb poles. If we restructure the jobs we won't have people with the capability." There are a lot of issues and a lot of options being considered at this point. Developing special equipment for women is not necessarily discriminatory towards men. When we redesigned the staplegun used to fasten wire to a house, we considerably reduced the average force necessary to operate it, which put it in a much more reasonable range for women. But an improvement such as that makes it easier for males too.

**Richard H. Egdahl:** Do you have a double-edged sword? On one hand a consent decree says that you have to take very creative actions to change jobs so they are more available to women. On the other hand even though your statistics are improving, there are still more injuries and potential legal liability as a result.

**Reilly:** As far as I know, we have never been sued in a class action for the fact that women are having more injuries. We do get into workers' compensation of course and there is certainly a differential effect there. The consent decree has expired and negotiations are under way to come up with some new agreement between the Bell System and the government with respect to our affirmative action program. I don't yet know what direction that will take, but the issue of the higher accident rate and legal liability will certainly be raised, and resolved somehow.

**Donna J. Morrison:** What happens when a woman tries to qualify as a pole climber and your tests show that she would be physically unable to handle the job? Do you do further testing to determine whether she has the skills for another type of job, or do you just refuse her employment on the basis of the physical abilities test?

**Reilly:** It would depend on the openings in the company. The women would have the same opportunities as anyone else coming into the office. Much of our flow right now is within the company so we're getting a lot of women who are operators, for example, applying for outside jobs. They have other options, too—inside craft work or service representative positions. It so happens that the outside craft jobs right now are the ones where there is growth.

**Morrison:** Does the outside work pay better?

**Reilly:** No, the outside and inside are parallel.

**Morrison:** And do you have placement counselors to work with the women?

**Reilly:** The Employment Office or upgrade and transfer bureau is where applicants would be given information on the complete range of job options. Each job requires passing some kind of paper-and-pencil test. Our physical test is a last stage cutoff used only for the outside craft job requiring pole climbing. But, yes, they would certainly be advised of all the options available.

# Social Conditioning and the Culture of the Corporation

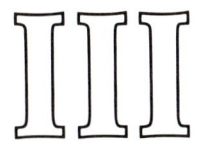

# III

# Changing Roles and Mental Health in Women

Jean F. Duff

# 5

Women participation in the labor force has increased substantially over the last thirty years. More than half of all women now work, and most work full-time. Further, more than half of all mothers work, and more divorced women work than women of other marital statuses.

From 1950 to 1975 female civilian labor force participation rate increased from 33.9 to 46.3 percent. From 1960 to 1970 the number of women in the civilian labor force as a percentage of the female civilian population increased from 50.1 to 54.3 percent.[1] By 1976, well over half the 47.3 million husband-and-wife families in the United States had more than one wage earner. As a result, nearly half of the children had mothers who were working or looking for work.[2] Female heads of households—about 7.5 million families in 1976[3]—have even higher labor force participation rates. Seventy-two percent of the 4 million divorced women were in the labor force in March 1975, compared with 55 percent of the 3 million separated women and 44 percent of the 47.5

million married women living with their husbands. Divorced women with children are also more likely than separated or married mothers to be in the work force.[4]

A great majority of female workers now work full-time. Sum's analysis of labor force participation indicates that "a substantial fraction of the rise in the female civilian labor force participation rate has been accounted for by an increase in the mean number of weeks spent in the labor force . . . (this) suggests that the temporary withdrawal rate (for childbearing and other family-related reasons) is being reduced in magnitude over time." [5]

This can be accounted for in a number of ways: the declining birth rate and more women's inclination to take short maternity leaves and return to work are two. Some women start careers or reenter the work force after children's earliest years. Estimates of the number of women reentering the labor force after several years absence for childrearing are difficult to obtain. Many older women are, however, seeking further education. In October 1976, of the 1.6 million people 35 years and over who were enrolled in school, 60 percent were women. Of these women, 65 percent were married. Sixty percent of the married women were also in the labor force as compared with 74 percent "not married" women in school.[6] Young notes that almost all the increase in enrollment among older women is accounted for by white, "not married" women—many of whom are self-supporting and may regard further education as necessary for career development.

## Women and Mental Health

Mental health can usefully be thought of in terms of personal competence. Personal competence implies a sense of mastery and control, or what Bandura[7] would term "self efficacy," and particularly capabilities for coping with life situations. Although the predictive value of the relationship remains unclear,[8] it is known that certain variables foster the development and maintenance of personal competence, while other variables threaten it. Among these are social supports, stressful events, and coping style.

### Variables Affecting Mental Health

Rachelle Warren clearly defines "social networks," the vehicle for social support:

> Social networks, or helping networks, refer to the various individuals each of us turns to for coping with daily and more serious problems of living. They are not groups. They often do not know each other. They are a combination of people we turn to in helping to solve a problem: a spouse, a neighbor, friends, relatives and

coworkers. Together they form the "natural helping networks" of an individual.[9]

People with few sources of social support are more vulnerable to stress than those who have the problem-solving and supportive resources of a "natural helping network" to draw upon.

Geographic mobility, increasing divorce and separation rates, the declining influence of church and community structures, as well as other aspects of social change, mean that all people are more at risk of losing social support. Women may have an additional vulnerability. For example, nearly 20 percent of all Americans move every year, disrupting family and friendship ties. Such moves may be more stressful to women than men since they are most often initiated by the men for employment advancement and may therefore be experienced by them as positive.[10]

Stressful life events, often a loss or disruption of social supports, have been shown to be associated with increased rates of physical and mental illness.[11] These events require adaptation to change, which may in some cases be beyond the capacity of the individual. Caplan[12] and others have shown that a crisis may either precipitate existing vulnerabilities, or, if handled successfully, may be an opportunity for mastery and growth.

Women have a special vulnerability to certain life events. Those associated with the reproductive cycle are specific to females, of course, and other events may have a particular significance for women as, for example, in the case of the economic implications of separation, divorce, or widowhood for a woman with young children. Finally, certain events have a greater frequency for women: in 1976, 12.4 percent of all females were widows compared with 2.7 percent of all men (data are standardized for age) (*Statistical Abstracts of the US 1977*, table 48).[13] However, despite these differences, several studies found no overall sex differences in the number of stressful life events reported,[14,15] although women consistently reported about 25 percent higher symptom intensities than men.

Coping style refers to the way a person deals with the anxiety associated with stress or change. Lazarus[16] distinguishes between adaptive and maladaptive reactions to stress and change and also divides the mechanisms into long-term and short-term. Long-term maladaptive coping results in physical or mental exhaustion, for example. Very little is known to date about normal patterns of coping among adults, although a new measure[17] which draws upon work by Green[18] is expected to yield interesting normative data.

Women tend to report more symptoms. Clancy and Gove[19] conclude that these are actual differences and not an artifact of response bias—women actually experienced more symptoms. Women predominate in every measure of utilization of the general health care system[20] and seek help at all levels more often than men.

Coping behaviors are learned and can be modified. Much has been written[21] about the "learned helplessness" syndrome in women—in effect a loss of confidence in ability to cope or a pattern of avoidance. This will be discussed further in the following section on depression because of the hypothesized causal relationship between the two.

Adequate social support, a low level of stressful events, and the presence of adaptive coping styles are associated with mental health in women. The syndrome most commonly associated with lack of mental well-being in women is depression.

## Depression in Women

Rates of depression among women, as measured in institutional and outpatient samples and in community surveys, consistently exceed those of men. Weissman and Klerman, in their review of sex differences and the epidemiology of depression, suggest that "by virtue of evolutionary selection, historical changes and social training, women are more sensitized to those psychosocial changes which disrupt attachment bonding and are therefore more vulnerable to depression."[22]

Higher rates of depression are found among women who are married and who have children living with them; older women whose children have left home and women who never married show fewer symptoms of depression.[23] Brown and others in a community survey found that working class women living at home with young children had the highest rates of depression—five times more than their middle class counterparts subject to equivalent levels of stress. Four factors contribute to this class difference: loss of a mother in childhood; three or more children under 14 living at home; absence of an intimate and confiding relationship with husband or boyfriend; lack of full-time or part-time employment outside of home. The first three factors were more frequent among working class women.[24] Interestingly, marriage appears to have a protective effect for men: rates of distress are highest for unmarried men and lowest for married men.

Some researchers argue strongly for the relationship between sex role stereotyping, in the form of learned helplessness in women, and the prevalence of depression among them. Seligman[25] defines "helplessness" as lack of control over rewards and punishments, and suggests in a recent article that "helplessness" can lead to "perceived helplessness" or a generalized belief that "nothing I do matters." This is likely to lead to depression, especially in the presence of stressful life events and the absence of protective resources. There is research evidence of a sex difference in both actual and perceived helplessness.

Jacquelyn Hall[26] in recent testimony before the Senate Committee on Human Resources further suggests that the unequal treatment that women receive in everyday life reinforces their sense of helplessness. Hall thus views the resulting depression as a public health problem derived from social and economic inequality.

In summary, then, it seems that disruption of social supports and loss of attachment bonds, coping styles based on avoidance and associated with feelings of helplessness, stressful life events, and women's rising expectations are all risk indicators of depression. These stressors may well have a greater impact on women because of their more vulnerable social position.[27]

## Work and Mental Health

Freud did not have women in mind when he gave his prescription for positive mental health, "love and work," but his advice does appear to hold true for women. With women participating in the labor force in ever greater numbers regardless of marital status and young children, both the protective and the stressful aspects of work for mental health assumes greater importance.

Employment outside the house may have a protective effect by alleviating boredom, increasing self-esteem, expanding social networks, and improving family finances. Women employed at low-level jobs, especially women with small children, are at high risk for depression, but women who are not employed show more symptoms of stress than working women.[28,29] The precise nature of the relationship between working and self-esteem and distress is difficult to assess because, since women have increasingly greater freedom to select the working role, the protective effect, if any, of working becomes obscured by self-selection. Women under greater stress at home may be more likely to seek out employment to relieve it. Thus two recent studies comparing work satisfaction of females with full-time employment and full-time housekeeping[30,31] both found few differences in attitudes toward self and in the degree of personal satisfaction.

The mental health of both working and nonworking women is vulnerable to the stressful effects of changing women's roles and especially of role conflict.

## Changing Roles and Role Conflict

A role is a set of expectations about how one should behave in a given situation. Traditional roles for women have been daughter, wife, mother, and widow. In these roles, the woman is usually defined in relation to another—even as a widow, a woman's role, and very often her status in society, has been defined in terms of her late husband. More recently the roles of worker, provider and single parent, and woman living alone have become available to women. Women moving into these new roles and combinations of them lack models or examples of how they should behave. They also lack clearly defined expectations for performance, and consequently frequently encounter difficulty in evaluating the degree to which they are performing the roles well.

## Types and Sources of Conflict

Role conflict, this difficulty in conforming to role expectations,[32] is associated with stress, low self-esteem, and depression.[33] It is useful to distinguish between intra- and interpersonal conflicts. The former might be experienced by a woman today who is caught in a period of social change where role definitions lack specificity and where the utility of existing role models is limited. Weissman and coworkers in an article on the educated housewife suggest that new role expectations may create these intrapsychic conflicts, particularly for those women who are involved in traditional family tasks but who also desire employment and recognition outside the family.[34] Fear of success, which we will refer to again later, is a manifestation of intrapersonal role conflict. Even for educated and economically comfortable women, ambivalence and conflict continue about roles, personality characteristics and occupations not traditionally seen as feminine.

Interpersonal conflict refers to a discrepancy between role expectations and role behavior. A woman who is trying to perform several roles at once, such as provider, mother, and wife, might well experience conflict as she tries to satisfy multiple sets of expectations and multiple needs. Few women today have role models in their own mothers or family members for dealing with the demands of multiple roles; they must find ways to reduce conflict by trial and error.

There is a strong tendency for women to place their own needs below those of others—in the case of mothers, below those of their husbands or their children—and to meet their own needs through extraordinary effort only after others' needs are met.[35] Conflict about roles, their priorities, and their satisfactory execution is almost inevitable.

Neville and Damico[36] in a study of role conflict among married women identified eight of the most common loci of interpersonal conflict.

conflict about time management
conflict about relations with husband

conflict about household management
conflict about financial matters
inward conflict
conflict with others
conflict about child care
conflict about expectations for self
conflict about expectations for others

Working women, and working mothers in particular, face particular sets of problems associated with performing multiple roles:

*Housework:* Many American women work two shifts in 24 hours because housework remains largely "women's work."

*Child care:* Fewer than 1 percent of the children of working mothers are in group day care centers.[37] The United States falls far behind other countries in the provision of child care facilities, this despite the many studies of the effects of day care on children which have indicated no adverse effects.[38] If role conflict is to be minimized and the economic role of women maximized, then, as Judith Brown suggests, either their responsibilities in child care must be reduced or the economic activity must be receptive, interruptible, not dangerous, and close to home.[39]

*Financial pressures:* Equal opportunity programs and affirmative action notwithstanding, qualified women employed full-time in 1976 earned less than 56 percent of what men earned, whereas in 1967 women's earnings were 62 percent of men's. One woman in four, but one man in eighteen, lives on less than $4,000 a year. Female heads of households are especially vulnerable, having a comparatively low family income.[40]

*Occupational inequality:* Because of a woman's reproductive and maternal roles, some employers expect a lack of continuity in a woman's career.[41] This attitude becomes a self-fulfilling prophecy when employers are reluctant to risk hiring a woman for positions that require a substantial commitment and time investment from the employee. Underutilized, bored employees of both sexes have higher turnover rates. While the proportion of women in the major professions has risen dramatically, they are still disproportionately represented in low paying, dead-end jobs.[42] One study of sex discrimination using a simulation network found that women were hired as frequently as identically qualified males, but were offered a lower starting salary and were offered second-year raises that increased the salary discrepancy between the sexes.[43]

Both economic and occupational inequality contribute to low self-esteem and to role conflict among women.

## Sex Role Stereotypes

Roles have tended to be strongly linked to sex-specific behavior. Rosencrantz[44] defines sex role stereotypes as "consensual beliefs about the differing characteristics of men and women in our society." Role conflict, both intra- and interpersonal, arises for women with perceived violations of what is considered "feminine." Women have tended to tailor their goals so as to minimize such conflict. Thus, Parsons et al.[45] found that there was an inverse relationship between traditional sex role values and the aspiration to achieve in education, income, and work plans.

Some theorists have suggested that fear of success in women curbs achievement. L. W. Hoffman[46,47] made a follow-up study of Horner's[48] original construct by readministering the fear of success measure to Horner's original subjects after ten years. Hoffman hypothesized that if fear of success reflected a conflict in which success signifies affiliative loss and failure as a woman, then women with this fear might be expected to marry and have children sooner. They did both. Results also supported the hypothesis that women with higher scores on the fear of success measure more often became pregnant when faced with success relative to their husbands. Pregnancy removes the woman from the achievement area, confirms her femininity, and reestablishes an affiliative relationship with her husband.

Interestingly, the recent literature on sex differences in achievement motivation indicates that no real differences have been demonstrated.[49] In a study by M. L. Hoffman[50] of both children and adults, males were found to value achievement more, although other research indicates that females are as likely as males to have achievement motives aroused in situations that call for achievement and do not conflict with other values.

## Role Stereotyping and Learned Helplessness

Sex role stereotyping in the form of "learned helplessness" is clearly related to low self-esteem in women. The similarity between the self-concept of women and their feminine stereotype, together with women's agreement with the greater social desirability of masculine traits, led Rosencrantz et al.[51] to conclude that women hold negative values of their own worth relative to men. Since 1968, however, significant changes have had an impact on women's self-concept.

It may well be that sex differences in the "learned helplessness" phenomenon will die out as the loss of women's power from the decline in importance of traditional family structure and roles is offset by the increasing opportunities for mastery available to women in the workplace and elsewhere. In such a context, a reduction of the high rate of depression among women would, Weissman and Klerman suggest, be indirect confirmation of the hypothesis that the female excess of depression is due to the disadvantages of the female role.

Little is known as yet about the relationship between feelings of personal competence and powerfulness (including the converse of "helplessness") and actual performance. One study of personal characteristics differentiating female executives from female nonexecutive personnel[52] found that executives had higher scores on the self-esteem component of the needs achievement measure, as well as higher levels of power motivation and mental ability than their nonexecutive counterparts.

A sense of mastery, or perceived effectiveness of performance, is thought to depend on the extent to which persons attribute their success or failure to internal factors such as their own ability or effort, rather than to external factors of task difficulty or luck.[53,54] The conditions associated with an increase in sense of mastery and personal competence as a result of job performance are worthy of further study.

## Changing Sex Role Stereotyping

The trends in today's society toward smaller families, white collars, increased education of women, and increased participation of women in economic activities all tend to accelerate the rate of change of sex role behaviors. In a study[55] of 1,400 women in management positions, only 10 percent identified sex-related difficulties as their greatest ones. Most problems cited were traditional ones including training opportunities and opportunities for advancement, experienced by men and women alike.

Women, especially those in supervisory positions, tend to have fewer sources of social support than their male counterparts. This is important because of the buffer effect that social support appears to have on stress. Baron's study[56] indicated that 25 percent of the women surveyed felt excluded from the more informal training and guidance that male executives normally provide to younger managers. These findings are in keeping with those of an earlier study by Epstein[57] of women in the professions. She found that structured professional processes in addition to the sponsor-protegé relationship, such as the colleague system and social interactions within organizations, cause the sex status of women to equal or surpass their occupational status as factors in the progress of women's careers.

A study of women who work in occupations generally considered appropriate to men reveals that while they enjoy the increased earnings, they do encounter some discrimination on the job.[58] According to Oppenheimer,[59] three factors tending in 1968 to keep certain jobs predominantly male were: career continuity (because career continuity and skills development are likely to be interrupted by women's family life cycle); motivation (being secondary breadwinners and primary family caretakers, women are not expected to have the career motivation of men); and geographic mobility (careers involving geographic mobility are closed to women who give priority to their husband's career). Just over ten years later, we see changes in rates of labor force participation and different reasons for women working. Career continuity is higher—most female workers work full-time; motivation is high—many female workers are either head of household or contributing an essential portion of the family income; and the relocation of women employees and their families is as much a topic of discussion as the geographic mobility of their men.

There is increasing evidence that traditional sex role socialization may not be conducive to adjustment by either sex. M. L. Hoffman, in a review of the literature, highlights some of the implications of sex role socialization for men today:

> The trend toward de-differentiation of sex roles may pose more problems for males than females. The new challenge for girls to develop and sustain individual achievement goals does not introduce a radically new motive for most of them, nor does it require them to change previously developed motives since their early schooling trained them to compete, achieve, and use their individual competencies. Besides, in the emerging post industrial era, the emphasis is shifting from production and technical skills to manipulation of words and ideas and interacting with people, skills similar to those involved in traditional female socialization. The challenge is greater for males because they are increasingly expected to contribute their share to the more "expressive" side of family and social life. This implies the expression of motives and interests that may well have been forcefully socialized out of them in childhood. Traditional masculine socialization may thus be a particular handicap for boys growing up during this period of cultural transition.
>
> Androgenous socialization then may best equip people to handle changing role demands through the life cycle. And the roles themselves may also become less stereotyped as they are increasingly filled by androgenous individuals.[60] (P. 315.)

There is evidence to support a relationship between dedifferentiation of sex roles and work competence. Bachtold and Werner,[61] in a study of successful women in biology and chemistry, found that their composite profile on a personality test was strikingly similar to that of men in biology and physics. Since their profile also differed markedly from that of either men or women in the general population, the authors concluded that there is a generalized "scientist" personality profile that is not determined by sex.

Although performance of work roles may be increasingly free of influences associated with sex role stereotypes, there is ample evidence to suggest that the evaluation of potential and performance continues to determine these stereotypes. Rosen and Jerdee,[62] in a survey of subscribers to the *Harvard Business Review*, document the potential for differential treatment of men and women in such work areas as selection, training, promotion, and career development. See also Korman's review of personnel attitudes and motivation.[63]

The effects of such restrictions on women's mental health are difficult to assess. Several writers have suggested that a generalized inequality in the treatment of women may render a woman more vulnerable to stress.[64,65,66] It is undoubtedly true that the movement of women into more significant positions at work will be greatly hampered by the inappropriate role stereotypes which men and women have of each other and of themselves, and by the tendency to act in a manner consistent with these stereotypes.[67]

## Conclusion

As the stereotypes for feminine behavior become less rigid, woman's mental health can be expected to benefit from changes in her own expectations as well as those of others. If the projections of Weissman and others are correct, such changes may be reflected in decreasing rates of depression among women. We can also expect, however, to see women turning to coping styles traditionally used by men. Weissman and Klerman[68] suggest some indications that this may now be occurring in that female rates of alcoholism, suicide, and crime have begun to rise.

Certain very significant steps need to be taken in the work site to reduce stress and bolster mental health for women. Movement toward the elimination of sex-linked inequities in reimbursement and advancement will work to reduce the associated intrapersonal conflict. Any means that can be found to ease the burden of dual roles for working mothers (help in locating or financing child care, flex-time, etc.) will act to reduce the interpersonal conflicts discussed earlier.

Increasingly, employees will be considering the health of their entire work force, regardless of sex. Betty Friedan, that bastion of women's liberation, in giving testimony in recent congressional hearings concerning women's midlife crises, disagreed with preceding speakers who called for special programs for women:

> With the increased burden on all our tax dollars, I do not think we can realistically expect such programs for women even if today's mid-life women are facing more stringent economic problems because of obsolete or inadequate preparation for mid-life and beyond. Both men and women need new kind of tax credits, low interest loans, educational subsidies, and counseling in their mid-life crises—and both men and women need new options of flex-time, part-time, shared jobs, ... low interest loans ... the kind of options government policies make available now only to the young.[69]

We look forward to the day when the major thrust of efforts to promote mental health in the worksite can be focused on problems shared by the sexes rather than on problems that differentiate them.

---

## NOTES

1. Andrew M. Sum, "Women in the Labor Force: Why Projections Have Been Too Low," *Monthly Labor Review* 100 (July 1977): 18–24.
2. Janet Norwood, "New Approaches to Statistics on the Family," *Monthly Labor Review* 100 (July 1977): 31–34.
3. Ibid.
4. Allyson Sherman Grossman, "The Labor Force Patterns of Divorced and Separated Women," *Monthly Labor Review* 100 (January 1977): 48–53.
5. Sum, "Women," p. 23.
6. Anne McDougall Young, "Going Back to School at 35 and Over," *Monthly Labor Review* 100 (July 1977): 43–45.
7. Albert Bandura, "Self-Efficacy: Toward a Unifying Theory of Behavioral Change," *Psychological Review* 84 (1977): 191–215.
8. A. A. Goetz, J. D. Duff, and J. B. Bernstein, "Health Risk Appraisal: The Estimation of Risk," in DHEW, Office of Health Information and Health Promotion, National Conference on Health Promotion, *Programs in Occupational Settings: State-of-the-Art Papers*, Washington, D.C., January 1979.
9. R. B. Warren, Paper prepared for Presidential Commission, 1977 (See under Report to the President): 1080.
10. M. M. Weissman, and E. S. Paykel, "Moving and Depression in Women," *Society* 9 (1972): 24–28.
11. Judith Godwin Rabkin and Elmer L. Struening, "Social Change, Stress and Illness: A Selective Literature Review," *Psychoanalysis and Contemporary Science* 5 (1976): 573–624.
12. G. Caplan, *Principles of Preventive Psychiatry* (New York: Basic Books, 1964).

13. *Statistical Abstracts of the United States*, 1977: Table 48.
14. E. H. Uhlenhuth and E. S. Paykel, "Symptom Configuration and Life Events," *Archives of General Psychiatry* 28 (1973): 744–748.
15. E. H. Uhlenhuth and E. S. Paykel, "Symptom Intensity and Life Events," *Archives of General Psychiatry* 28, (1973): 473–477.
16. R. S. Lazarus, *Psychological Stress and the Coping Process* (New York: McGraw-Hill, 1966).
17. General Health, Inc., *Personal Health Profile* (Washington, D.C.: 1979).
18. L. W. Green, I. Figa-Talamancea, H. Kalmer, G. D. Mellinger, and D. I. Manheimer, "Self-Care Patterns of Normal Adults in Response to Mild Symptoms of Stress," Paper presented to American Public Health Association, Miami, Fla., October 18, 1976.
19. K. Clancy and W. Gove, "Sex Differences in Mental Illness: An Analysis of Response Bias in Self-Reports," *American Journal of Sociology* 80 (1974): 205–216.
20. M. M. Weissman and G. Klerman, "Sex Differences and the Epidemiology of Depression," in *Gender and Disordered Behavior: Sex Differences in Psychopathology*, ed. Edith S. Gomberg and Violet Franks (New York: Brunner Mazel, 1979).
21. M. E. Seligman, "Depression and Learned Helplessness," in *The Psychology of Depression: Contemporary Theory and Research*, ed. R. J. Friedman, and M. M. Katz (Washington, D.C.: Winston, 1974).
22. Weissman et al., "Sex Differences," p. 417.
23. Weissman et al., "Sex Differences."
24. G. Brown, M. Bhrolchain, and T. Hariss, "Social Class and Psychiatric Disturbance among Women in an Urban Population," *Sociology* (1975): 225–254.
25. Seligman, "Depression."
26. Hearings on "The Coming Decade; Women and Human Resources," *Congressional Information Services Index* 7 (ref. 5541–6), (July 1979): 581–703.
27. G. L. Klerman, "Depression and Adaptation," in *The Psychology of Depression*.
28. L. S. Radloff, "Sex Differences in Depression: The Effects of Occupation and Marital Status," *Sex Roles* 1 (1975): 249–265.
29. Brown et al., "Social Class."
30. L. W. Hoffman and F. J. Nye, *Working Mothers* (San Francisco: Jossey-Bass, 1974).
31. C. N. Weaver and F. L. Holmes, "Comparative Study of Work Satisfaction of Females with Full-time Employment and Full-time Housekeeping," *Journal of Applied Psychology* 60 (1975): 117–118.
32. Dorothy Nevill and S. Damico, "Role Conflict in Women as a Function of Marital Status," *Human Relations* 28 (1975): 487–497.
33. M. M. Weissman, C. Pincus, and B. Prosoff, "The Educated Housewife: Mild Depression and the Search for Work," *American Journal of Orthopsychiatry* 43 (1973): 565–573.

## Social Conditioning and the Culture of the Corporation

34. Ibid.
35. Celia M. Halas, "Sex-Role Stereotypes: Perceived Childhood Socialization Experiences and the Attitudes and Behaviors of Mature Women," *Dissertation Abstracts International* 35 (1974): 1499A.
36. Neville and Damico, "Role Conflict."
37. Report to the President from the President's Commission on Mental Health: "Report of the Special Populations Sub-panel on Mental Health of Women," III, Appendix (Washington, D.C.: U.S. Government Printing Office, 1978): 1022–1116.
38. J. E. Chapman and J. B. Lazar, *Review of Present Status and Future Needs in Day Care Research*, monograph (Washington, D.C.: George Washington University Press, 1971).
39. Judith K. Brown, "A Note on the Division of Labor by Sex," *American Anthropologist* 72 (1970): 1074–1078.
40. Grossman, "The Labor Force."
41. Valerie Kincade Oppenheimer, "The Sex Labeling of Jobs," *Industrial Relations* 7 (1968): 219–234.
42. Report of the National Commission on the Observance of International Women's Year (1976).
43. J. R. Terborg and D. R. Ilgen, "A Theoretical Approach to Sex Discrimination in Traditional Masculine Occupations," *Organizational Behavior and Human Performance* 13 (1975): 352–376.
44. P. S. Rosenkrantz, S. R. Vogel, H. Bee, I. K. Broverman, and D. M. Broverman, "Sex Role Stereotypes and Self-Concepts in College Students," *Journal of Consulting and Clinical Psychology* 32, (1968): 287–295.
45. J. E. Parsons, I. H. Frieze, D. Ruble, and J. Croke, "Intrapsychic Factors Influencing Career Aspirations in College Women," unpublished, 1975. Quoted in President's Commission on Mental Health Report III (1978): 1061.
46. L. W. Hoffman, "Fear of Success in Males and Females, 1965 and 1972," *Journal of Consulting and Clinical Psychology* 42 (1974): 353–358.
47. L. W. Hoffman, "Fear of Success in 1965 and 1974: A Follow-Up Study," *Journal of Consulting and Clinical Psychology* 45 (1976): 310.
48. M. Horner, "Towards an Understanding of Achievement Related Conflicts in Women," *Journal of Social Issues* 28 (1972): 157–175.
49. E. E. Maccoby and C. N. Jacklin, Psychology of Sex Differences (Palo Alto: Stanford University Press, 1974).
50. M. L. Hoffman, "Sex Differences in Moral Internalization and Values," *Journal of Personality and Social Psychology* 32 (1975): 720–729.
51. Rosenkrantz et al., "Sex Role Stereotypes."
52. R. F. Morrison and M. C. Sebald, "Personal Characteristics Differentiating Female Executives from Female Non-Executive Personnel," *Journal of Applied Psychology* 59 (1974): 656–659.
53. B. Weiner, "Achievement Motivation As Conceptualized by an Attribution Theorist," in *Achievement Motivation and Attribution Theory*, ed. B. Weiner (Morristown, N.J.: General Learning Press, 1974): 3–48.

54. A. K. Korman, "Hypothesis of Work Behavior Revisited and an Extension," *Academic Management Review* 1 (1976): 50–63.
55. Alma Baron, "Women in Management: A New Look," *Personnel Administration* (December 1978).
56. Ibid.
57. Cynthia Fuchs Epstein, "Encountering the Male 'Establishment': Sex Status Limits on Women's Careers in the Professions," *American Journal of Sociology* 75 (1970): 965–982.
58. L. Walshok, "Nontraditional Blue Collar Work among Urban Women" (San Diego: Univ. of California extension, NIMH Grant #R01 MH27685).
59. Oppenheimer, "Sex Labeling."
60. M. L. Hoffman, "Personality and Social Development," *Annual Review of Psychology* 28 (1977): 295–321.
61. Louise M. Bachtold and Emmy E. Werner, "Personality Characteristics of Women Scientists," *Psychological Reports* 31 (1972): 391–396.
62. B. Rosen and T. H. Jerdee, "Sex Stereotyping in the Executive Suite," *Harvard Business Review* 52 (1974): 45–58.
63. A. K. Korman, J. H. Greenhaus, and I. J. Badin, "Personnel Attitudes and Motivation," *Annual Review of Psychology* 28 (1977): 175–196.
64. Klerman, "Depression and Adaptation."
65. Weissman et al., "Educated Housewife."
66. Hearings on "The Coming Decade."
67. V. E. O'Leary, "Some Attitudinal Barriers to Occupational Aspirations in Women," *Psychological Bulletin* 81 (1974): 809–826.
68. Weissman et al., "Sex Differences."
69. Judy Mann, "Society's Next Frontier: Solving Mid-life Demands," *Washington Post* (May 9, 1979).

## Discussion

**Jean F. Duff:** I wish we had the hard data on the behavioral considerations that AT&T brought to bear on the pole-climbing program. We don't. But there are some things we know. There is evidence to suggest that work—a generalization here—seems to be good for women's mental health. We know that women who are at highest risk of mental illness are women with children under six, married women who are not working, and women who suffer from some of the stresses associated with poverty. Subsets of those groups who are working seem to have lower rates of mental illness of one kind or another. The issue of sexual stereotyping is critical. There are not unique stresses in the workplace that impinge upon women but rather a conflict between expectations of self and expectations of others, especially men, regarding the role performance of women. And we're looking at, among other things, a learning situation, without adequate role models. Sexual stereotype problems impinge on self-esteem, performance, and progression up the corporate ladder. Otherwise, the principal stresses on women seem to relate to role conflict and a set of problems posed by childrearing and trying to balance that with career goals.

**Kenneth C. Edelin:** Let me make the provocative statement that if industry had its complete freedom of choice, it would prefer not to hire young women, basically because of the biological differences having to do with reproduction. When you hire young women, they either already have a family and family obligations that perhaps will increase their absenteeism, or the possibility remains that they will decide to start a family and therefore disrupt the continuity of work to take maternity leave. The real truth may be that if employers had their druthers, they would not choose women, and that's why women are finding it so difficult not only to enter the work force but also to move up the corporate ladder. If industry really wanted to, it could adapt jobs to accommodate the individual differences among us all as far as physical capabilities are concerned.

**Eleanor Tilson:** It is true that absenteeism among women is not so much related to illness as to the lack of adequate child care. Child care is the key to this issue.

**Nina G. Stillman:** Some studies that have been done among women attorneys indicate that as women enter the professions, they are taking much less time off for child care than traditionally might have been expected. We found in Chicago that when women attorneys have children, many are away from work only two to three weeks. Very rarely did we have six weeks. This may have to do with the level of interest and involvement in the job and of course the economic factor that they can afford high-quality child care.

**Robert M. Clyne:** Dr. Edelin is probably right that most any job could be engineered for most any person, male, female, even children if the child labor laws allowed it. But the question I would pose is can we as a society afford everything that we are talking about doing? The producer, the manufacturer, is only a middle man. If he cannot pass along the cost to the consumer, he goes out of business. But in these inflationary times are we willing to pay five dollars for a loaf of bread in order to pay for modifications in the production process? That's something we have to decide: Can we afford it? Can we be competitive in the world? It isn't just a social question, it's a question of economics and survival.

**Jeanne M. Stellman:** I submit that our inflation worries today are in no way related to whatever inroads equal opportunity has made. I don't think, for example, that low productivity of women workers in the oil industry has in any way caused the rise in the price of petroleum products which is probably the major contributor to inflation in the overall economy right now.

**Duff:** I would push a step further and suggest the controversial opinion that perhaps some of the very extensive steps that some industries are taking on behalf of women are not only contributing to the expense of services and products, as Dr. Clyne suggests, but also inadvertantly contributing to a diminution of the competence of the worker. I'd like to see the issue addressed in terms of how to make workers more competent to judge the stresses and the risks of working and the means of alleviating them. Just as employers have an obligation to inform workers about potential toxins and other health hazards in the workplace, I believe that we need more involvement of the worker and the prospective worker in assessing for him or herself the risks associated with starting employment or continuing employment under various circumstances.

# Employee Health Services for Women Workers*

Leon J. Warshaw

## 6

More than ever before and at a rate that has surpassed all projections, women are taking and keeping jobs outside the home. While they continue to concentrate in their traditional white collar and service jobs, increasing numbers are entering blue collar, craft, technical, and professional categories from which they had hitherto largely been excluded. The numbers of women working as laborers and in agriculture have also grown, along with female representation in supervisory and managerial positions. This movement has been part of a veritable social revolution marked by changing expectations of and attitudes toward the roles of women as workers, homemakers, bearers of children, and members of society.

These changes have presented particular challenges to occupational

*Reprinted from *Preventive Medicine Journal* **7**, 385–393 (Academic Press, N.Y., 1978) with permission of the publisher.

health professionals and have dictated modifications in the employee health programs for which they are responsible. This paper will attempt to outline three major aspects in which the modern comprehensive employee health service has adapted to the new roles of women*: job placement and the design of work tasks; the social structure and interpersonal relationships in the work group; and pregnancy.

## The Modern Employee Health Program

First, to view these in proper perspective, it seems advisable to reiterate that, to meet its fundamental objective of maintaining the health of the work force, the modern employee health program seeks to:

place each worker in a job that he/she can perform without endangering himself/herself, co-workers, or the public;

monitor job tasks and the work environment to identify materials and activities that might be harmful and recommend changes that would eliminate or satisfactorily control such hazards;

identify workers whose individual characteristics or prior work experiences make them especially susceptible to a particular occupational hazard and recommend appropriate steps to control it or to protect them from its influence;

recommend to management appropriate modifications in the organization of work, personnel relations, benefit programs, and workplace amenities that will enhance employee health and well-being;

provide educational and training programs to enable employees to recognize and cope with potential work hazards, and to encourage their acceptance of preventive health services and the adoption of healthful life styles; and

enhance the accessibility, availability, and quality of community health care resources and encourage their appropriate utilization by employees and their dependents.

Achievement of these goals has been complicated by growing awareness of and concern about the health effects of industrial products and processes. The traditional focus on accidents and acute poisoning has been broadened to cover the cumulative effects of repeated injuries, the subtle effects of chronic low-level exposures to

*It must be emphasized that these roles are "new" only in quantitative terms: they now represent so significant a percentage of the work force that they can no longer be dealt with on an *ad hoc* basis or completely ignored.

toxic agents, and the contribution of occupational and environmental exposures to such multifactorial diseases as cancer, myocardial infarction, and pulmonary insufficiency. It now also includes the impact on emotional health and social well-being of the organization of work and the interpersonal relationships in the workplace. Employers have been assuming increasing responsibility for eliminating or at least mitigating these effects reflecting both the enlightened self-interest implicit in their greater acceptance of today's concepts of corporate social responsibility and their compliance with the dictates of new laws, governmental regulations, and labor–management agreements. This is underscored by industry's awareness that healthy, well-functioning workers are more productive.

## Job Placement of Women

From early childhood on, boys outdo girls in activities requiring strength and/or speed while girls outperform boys in motor tasks requiring fine coordination and accuracy. As they grow, these differences become more pronounced. To some extent, they reflect cultural and social factors that, until recently, have emphasized athletics and physical tasks for boys while relegating girls to sedentary handwork activities. However, for the most part, they reflect basic differences in body structure and mechanics. On the average, adult men are about 25 percent heavier than adult women and, having more muscle tissue relative to body weight, possess greater strength, endurance, and power. This means that women cannot lift, hold, or carry as much weight; they cannot push or pull as heavy loads; their grips are not as strong; and they cannot exert as much force on a foot pedal.

In addition, the males' longer growth period results in greater standing and sitting height, longer arms and legs, larger hands and feet, and greater chest girth and breathing capacity. Since most machines, tools, and work benches are built to the scale of men, women are at an even greater disadvantage in performing physical work.

But these are generalizations. The range of variations among women overlaps that among men; i.e., some women are larger, stronger, and more physically capable than some men. Further, most jobs in industry are not very demanding in relation to the average individual's physical potentials, and many of those that are can often be made less demanding by modifying the job and/or redesigning the equipment it involves. This leaves only a very few jobs that require the intensity and level of physical effort that can be applied only by the physically gifted. Except for these, there appears to be no justification for the automatic exclusion of women from jobs requiring physical work.

The key is selective placement, a process developed decades ago to permit employment of the handicapped which is used in employee health programs to assure a proper fit between a potential worker and a particular job. This involves, first, an analysis of the job and the circumstances under which it is performed. This should be based on direct observation with proper allowance for tasks that are infrequently performed and any potential emergencies. Experience has amply demonstrated that job titles and stereotyped job descriptions are often misleading.

Next, the characteristics and capabilities of the worker are assessed. This may involve observation and a few simple tests or carefully calibrated measurements of strength, physical fitness, and aptitude. In most instances, the worker's capabilities can be enhanced by programs of physical conditioning and preliminary job training.

When these do not suffice, recommendations can be developed for redesigning the job or retooling it. Such changes are not inexpensive but experience in a number of industries has shown them to be economically sound. Not only have they made it possible to comply with regulations dictating the employment of women but they have increased the comfort, efficiency, and productivity of male workers.

## Environmental Hazards

Most of the present knowledge of potential environmental hazards is based on experience with men and experimental animals. However, except during pregnancy which will be discussed below, there appears to be no significant difference between men and women with respect to susceptibility to toxic environmental agents. If the working environment is safe for men, it should be equally safe for women.

In instances in which engineering technology cannot be applied to the control of environmental hazards, personal protective equipment and devices are employed to shield workers from their effects. Since these are usually sized to fit the male frame, they may not provide the desired protection for women. Poor fit can vitiate the protective effects of respirators and harnesses, while safety shoes and garments that are too large can precipitate accidents. Women may have to be temporarily barred from tasks that require the use of personal protective equipment until the medical director can locate a vendor who can provide the necessary items sized to fit them.

An axiom in the control of workplace hazards is that many can be eliminated simply by attention to good housekeeping. Care in stacking and storage of materials, frequent collection and proper disposal of waste and debris, prompt mop-up of spills and scatters, and routine cleanliness have been shown not only to eliminate potential hazards but also to enhance the quality of production. It has been observed that the addition of women to a work crew has been followed by improved housekeeping. This has been attributed to the insistence of the more fastidious women workers and also to primping on the part of the male workers as an implicit response to the "distaff" influence. Whatever the cause, such improvement in the workplace benefits both sexes.

## The Impact of Women in the Workplace

The impact of the introduction of women into formerly all-male work situations has been both exaggerated and understated. There have been instances in which the surfacing of deep-rooted and subtle emotional problems has been precipitated. At the same time (and sometimes involving the same people) there have been strident demands and posturing that, despite their alleged symbolic significance, have bordered on the ridiculous. Since emotional and behavioral difficulties can be no less disabling than physical injury and disease, since they can spread among a work group no less rapidly than chicken pox in a grade school class, and, because they can usually be relieved and often prevented, they receive major attention in the modern employee health program.

Prevention is best initiated by the issuing by top management of a simply worded policy statement that explicitly defines the attitudes and interpersonal behavior it expects in the workplace. The effect would be enhanced if any unions that may be involved would either endorse it or independently issue supportive statements. This policy should be emphasized and reiterated in all employee orientation and retraining programs. Periodic meetings of small groups of coworkers to discuss work assignments and performance can allow for the ventilation and defusing of problems that otherwise might be expressed in destructive behavior. Finally, one-to-one counseling can guide a potentially troubled employee to cope with these problems as they arise.

Secondary prevention involves the early identification of the person with emerging difficulty and taking appropriate steps to deal with it, not only for the benefit of that individual but also to control any adverse effects on other members of the work unit. The employee health staff is sensitized to the potential significance of somatic symptoms that are repeated or come in clusters. Managers and supervisors are trained to recognize the pattern of frequent tardiness and short-term absences, impaired work performance, changes in dress and appearance, and unusual behavior and to promptly refer those who exhibit it to the employee health service for evaluation and treatment. Finally, when the employee health service has earned a reputation for helpfulness, competence, and integrity, workers will voluntarily seek its help when they are troubled.

The preceding paragraphs have been deliberately written to be applicable to both sexes despite the general impression that women are more susceptible to emotional difficulties, odd behavior, and flightiness. That impression is substantiated by data indicating that women make more visits to mental health professionals and clinics, are more frequently tagged with a psychiatric diagnosis, and take more tranquilizers and other psychotropic medications. While such statistics have been repeatedly validated in the community, they do not seem to hold in the workplace. I have found neither the frequency nor the severity of mental illness to be greater among women than in their male co-workers.

Women, however, do seem to have more problems with their social adjustments to work. In part, this reflects the fact that so many married women workers continue to bear their traditional responsibilities for homemaking and the rearing of children. Also, there are many more unmarried, divorced, or widowed women with young children than single-parent households headed by men. These burdens are distracting, time-consuming, and fatiguing; they often lead not only to impaired work performance and absenteeism,* but to guilt, frustration, and dissatisfaction. Flextime or other modification of the work schedule is often uniquely beneficial; for example, it may permit a working mother to be at home when her child is out of school. In many instances—although still far too few—company- or union-sponsored day-care centers have attempted to make up for the lack of such facilities in the community.

In part, the woman worker's problems reflect the fact that she is a newcomer in the work group. As a colleague put it, "she doesn't know how to behave in that male locker room and the men don't quite know how to react to her presence." The aggressiveness that the woman had to muster to enter this domain and her justified resentment in instances when she had to be better qualified and accept lower pay to win the job are sometimes translated into an abrasiveness that makes her hard to take. For the men, her new presence sometimes shatters the cohesiveness of the work group from which some derive the social support that holds their daily lives together.

*It is noteworthy that, among policemen, firemen, and other uniformed municipal employees who enjoy unlimited sick leave with full pay and whose wives work at jobs with limited paid sick leave, it is the husband who reports "ill" and stays home to care for a sick child.

Although I believe that its importance is overstated, sexual behavior—real or only perceived—may present problems, e.g., female seductiveness and male machismo in dress, speech, and conduct and advances that are made, not made, or rejected. The propinquity dictated by certain jobs can cause problems either directly for the worker or by provoking jealousy in a susceptible spouse. This has occurred when a woman had to accompany a man on long business trips away from home and when a policewoman was assigned to spend her days cruising in a police car with her male partner. Such problems may simply require guidance in coping with outmoded mores. However, there are instances in which fundamental sexual "hang-ups" are exposed and more specific therapy is required.

The two-career family presents a different constellation of social problems. These range from such simple adjustments as sharing housework or coordinating vacation schedules to such extremely difficult dilemmas as when one career requires relocation to a distant locale where the other cannot flourish. Expert counseling is sometimes needed to prevent disruption of the marriage or, if that cannot be accomplished, to assist in coping with a divorce.

The point is that most of these emotional and social difficulties can be predicted if one knows the situation and the people involved in it. To learn what is happening or about to happen, the medical director maintains ongoing contacts with key company officials and close collaboration with the director of personnel and, at the same time, stays tuned in to the company grapevine. Appropriate intervention is initiated promptly by the employee health staff and, when necessary, their efforts are supplemented by prearranged resources procured by the organization or available in the community. In addition to assisting the individual worker to develop more effective adaptive and coping mechanisms, the medical director, recommends helpful changes in work groupings, schedules, and assignments; arranges suitable educational, indoctrination, and training programs for workers and supervisors; and guides management toward the adoption and implementation of policies and procedures that will make working a more healthful and rewarding experience. Although it is difficult to measure the many intangibles involved, it is my impression that such a program often yields a more favorable cost–benefit ratio than any of the other preventive health activities that might be pursued.

## Medical Problems Unique to Women

Gynecologic disorders, breast and pelvic cancer, and pregnancy require special attention in an employee health program serving women workers. Repeated surveys have shown that, when these are deleted from the statistics, the universally observed increased absenteeism of women drops to the same levels as those of men.

Menstrual irregularities, dysmenorrhea, and hypermenorrhea, and the secondary anemia that is its frequent concomitant, account for a large number of the visits logged by the employee health service and constitute a major cause of short-term absences and disability. Dysmenorrhea, for example, and/or the medications taken to relieve it produce drowsiness, weakness, slowed reaction time, and impaired coordination. These not only impair productivity but set the stage for accidents and injuries. It is astonishing how many women passively endure these symptoms and how often they are received with cavalier disdain when they do consult their physicians about them. In addition to providing analgesics and an opportunity to rest during acute episodes, the employee health staff promotes more serious consideration of the problem by the worker and her personal physician and offers advice about regimens that have proven useful in preventing much of the discomfort.

In the periodic examinations or health screening offered by many employee health services, special attention is usually paid to the early detection and proper treatment of breast and pelvic cancer. Because few organizations have a large enough female population to justify the installation of mammography and thermography equipment, breast examinations are usually limited to palpation and instruction in self-examination. Pap smears prepared by a nurse or the patient herself are usually sent to outside laboratories for examination. These programs are a valuable, convenient, and low-cost (to the woman) supplement to the cancer detection efforts of the health professionals and voluntary organizations in the community.

## Pregnancy

Toxic exposures during work may affect childbearing women and their offspring by:

> impairment of fertility and/or damage to germ cells resulting in fetal wastage and congenital defects (these, it has been learned recently, may also occur in men);
> mutagenesis and abnormal development of the fetus;
> interference with the essential physiology of pregnancy leading to abortion, premature delivery, or fetal injury;
> combination with pre-existing or coincidental medical problems to cause maternal illness or injury;
> excretion of chemicals in breast milk that may cause toxicity in the nursing infant;

transplacental carcinogenesis—with the demonstration of the linkage between the administration of diethylstilbestrol to pregnant women and the subsequent appearance of genital cancer in their daughters, it has been suggested that the recent rise in cancer in children may be due to chemical exposures during pregnancy.

These potential effects have been the focus of much recent attention reflecting growing awareness of the more subtle effects of toxic agents that can be encountered in the workplace and the increasing numbers of women of childbearing age entering jobs in which they may be exposed to them.

The vast majority—over 90 percent—of pregnant workers will have normal pregnancies and healthy children. The unfortunate outcomes in some of the remainder are attributable to a variety of factors: genetic diseases, maternal infections, drugs, excessive use of alcohol, etc. In most cases, however, the cause is not known; it is quite possible that occupational exposures may be involved in some. While admittedly imperfect statistics do not appear to demonstrate any increase in bad outcomes that can be associated with work-related factors, it is evident that appropriate preventive measures might obviate such an increase and might even reduce the number that now occur.

The principals of preventing harm to the pregnant worker and her fetus are outlined in a recently published report, *Guidelines on Pregnancy and Work,* produced under the aegis of the American College of Obstetricians and Gynecologists and the National Institute of Occupational Safety and Health.* They start with the premise that a "normal woman with a normal pregnancy and a normal fetus in a job presenting no greater hazards than those encountered in daily life in the community may continue to work without interruption until the onset of labor and may resume working several weeks after an uncomplicated delivery."

They then guide the physician to an evaluation of the worker's health status touching on the maternal problems that may cause complications and the physiologic alterations of pregnancy that may present difficulty.

Next, attention is focused on fetal development and the possibility that it might be impaired or impeded by work stresses or by chemicals that cross the placental barrier. Here, because they are far more significant threats than the chemicals encountered in most workplaces, special emphasis is given to drugs that may be prescribed for or taken by the worker.

---

*This book is available from ACOG Publications, Suite 2700, One East Wacker Drive, Chicago, Illinois 60601 for $3.00 per copy.

Finally, the guidelines focus on the job the worker performs and the potential hazards it may involve. A format is provided for inquiry into the details of the work tasks probing their intensity, duration, and pattern and exploring the potential of ill effects from either the work or the environment in which it is done. Incidentally, the guidelines advise a similar detailed inquiry into activities performed in the home, in the community, and in recreational pursuits since, for most workers, they present much greater hazards than those of the job.

Then, using the logic conceptualized in a simple algorithm, the physician is guided to an analysis of all of the variables to determine if the individual worker can continue on her particular job without undue risk to her and her fetus. The physician may suggest modifications of the job to control or eliminate a potential hazard or simply to contribute to her comfort and well-being. Most important, the physician is urged to communicate the recommendations and their rationale to the worker in a manner that will encourage her to accept and implement them.

The lack of precise information about toxic exposure of women was noted earlier. Unhappily, there is even less knowledge of the impact of such exposures on the pregnant worker and her fetus. At the same time, it appears that complete elimination of known or suspected toxic agents from the workplace may not always be possible or practical. Under what circumstances, then, is it safe for the pregnant worker to stay on the job and when should she be advised or required to leave it? Even if we did have satisfactory answers to this question—and we are far from them—the problem would not be solved. Many pregnancies are not planned, and women often do not know they are pregnant until at least 30 and sometimes 60 days after conception. During this period, the fetus is most vulnerable to damage by many of the toxic agents to be found in the workplace.

The ethical, moral, economic, social, and legal implications of this problem are currently being hotly debated. Until adequate scientific information becomes available, an arbitrary solution will have to be imposed that, perforce, will leave many unsatisfied. I am unable to predict what form it will take but would plead that, every time it is applied, the woman be fully informed and allowed to participate in the decisions that stem from it.

## Conclusion

The principles and procedures employed by the modern employee health service in serving the special needs of women workers are not new. But they need special emphasis as more women join the work force and take jobs from which they formerly were largely excluded. They also need the perfection that can come from research and carefully studied experience. They need expanded application not only in more and better employee health services but in the health care establishments in the community that serve women in industries without health services and those who are self-employed. Finally, if their ultimate purpose of maintaining health and well-being is to be achieved, they must be supplemented by changes in our social institutions to free the woman worker from the pervasive cultural biases that she now must endure.

## Discussion

**Jeanne M. Stellman:** I'd like to reinforce Dr. Warshaw's emphasis on social aspects of these problems. If we accept the fact that bearing and raising children is a social function and also accept the fact that we don't want the husband to stay home and become a wife so that women can move up the corporate ladder, then we need to restructure society. We need a "rediscover World War II" movement. Suddenly all the remedies appeared virtually overnight to enable women to go to work: child care, job sharing, and so on. It's bad enough that we live in a society that has deprived the fathers of raising their children. Do we now want to become a society where we deprive mothers of raising the children? Why not have a society where we have flexible jobs? Many professional couples that I know do similar work. I would not be adverse to sharing a job with my husband. That's my particular bias. The fact is that if we were to do such a thing we would both suffer professionally and economically. The United States is the only industrialized country without some form of system to deal with children and childbearing—absolutely the only one.

**Nina G. Stillman:** Work sharing comes up very frequently in the literature now. It makes some sense to the extent jobs are fungible. But in higher level jobs, moving into the executive decision-making area, or into medicine, it is not going to work. In a law practice, for example, if I go out of town for months at a time on a case, I can't suddenly in the middle of a trial tell whatever husband I might have that it's his turn. There are too many variables to be kept in mind that can't just be relayed to someone else at the appointed hour. Perhaps job sharing can work in a very mechanical type of job; where the husband knows how to build the tire and the wife knows how to build the tire, perhaps they can share in building it. But in any upper echelon job, there will be real problems. There will be some inescapable tradeoffs—if people opt for part-time work it will be at the expense of professional advancement.

**William J. Bicknell:** I tend to agree more with Jeanne Stellman. For instance in medicine, as in most occupations and professions, there is probably a lot more opportunity for job sharing than is commonly believed. Medicine may be different from law but no less complex, I suspect, and I believe that with a little creativity two physicians—husbands and wives or a couple living together—could work out a shared career. I recently talked to some partners in a major Boston law firm that has been grappling with this issue. They said the resistance was due much more to the value structure of the organization—protectiveness toward traditional roles and patterns—than to the very occasional instance where job sharing really does impinge upon critical decisions or getting the work done. It was clearly a wrenching thing for the upper echelon hierarchy of the law firm to consider. It was not so difficult for the firm to reorganize as difficult for the establishment to adjust to an alien value structure.

**Iver S. Ravin:** Are we in danger of substituting one stereotype of women for another? Some of us in my age group grew up with an image of women who played house when we played ball and took English literature while we took math and chemistry. Now we're finally liberating ourselves enough to adopt another image of women: a girl who in school is now taught that she doesn't have to be a nurse, she can be a doctor, or a lineworker, or be anything she wants, while boys are taught that it is all right to cook and stay home and take care of the kids. This is all to the good and some of us are now acclimated to this new image of women. She doesn't have to lose time for childbearing and childrearing. She can easily make the necessary arrangements for her children and when the kids get sick her husband can stay home. I wonder though. If we educate young girls today in this manner, free them from the necessity to stay home, then we as a society don't have to plan for the care and nurturing of their children—the women will handle that along with everything else—and we will perhaps end up with a new stereotype of a woman who can do everything that's at least as damaging as the old.

**Stellman:** I very much agree. I think we're creating a new image of superwoman which is a lot harder to live up to than the old. In the interest of equality, when we're assessing the broad health impact of professional work or line work or whatever kind of work on women, it is incumbent on us not to ignore the other side: the health costs to men of being deprived of family relationships, the demands of jobs and their impact on family life, the health costs of working till midnight, of leaving home before your children's breakfast, of having your children grow up without knowing who or what they are, of being transferred all around the country. What do these experiences mean in each of our lives? How much do we pay for them?

**Stellman:** I've read that IBM is finding that some men and their working wives have made the decision that success is not necessarily the be-all and end-all of existence. The company is finding that a lot of its bright young men just don't want to be moved from city to city after they have established roots and become involved in their community. As a result IBM is doing some serious rethinking as to whether they have to reevaluate the criteria for moving up the IBM ladder.

**Leslie I. Boden:** The fact that success is often in conflict with a decent family life is finally becoming clear now that men and women are both working. In the past the man could disengage from family life on a day-to-day basis, or uproot the family to move whenever necessary for his career. But now that both the man and the woman are out working, the tensions between job and family goals are much more clear.

As a result, some people are refusing to subordinate their roles as family members to their roles as employees. They may refuse promotions, relocations, or job offers. If many employees take such action, the corporations they work in may rethink whether people really have to move around to eight different cities in ten years in order to be good executives. I don't think anybody's ever done a study that demonstrates that current occupational mobility patterns in corporations or academia really produce better corporate executives or researchers or professors. It's never been looked at. The issue is just now surfacing because women and men are now both working.

# Special Needs of Women in Health Examinations

*Donna Morrison, R.N., Carmen Moynehan, Stanley P. deLisser, and William Wanago, M.D.*

# 7

### The "Man's World" of Health Exams

The present system of periodic health examinations does not adequately provide for female needs. A number of facts support this view. First, in the United States today, only 9.8 percent of all physicians are female, and of these, relatively few are in teaching positions. Medical textbooks published quite recently continue to describe women as passive, willing to suffer, self-sacrificing, and masochistic.[1] There is a general attitude among medical care providers that women are not able to make intelligent choices about treatment. Second, a survey by Executive Health Examiners (EHE) in 1975 found that 20 percent of the women interviewed felt that a periodic pelvic examination and Pap smear constituted an adequate check-up.

Another indicator that examinations are a man's world is in standard industry procedures. Not infrequently, exam programs in industry have breakpoints where the intensity of examination procedures or the frequency of examinations is increased. Most often these breakpoints are age-dictated, i.e., "up to age 40," "over age 55," etc. Although primarily budget motivated, these breakpoints are based on the presumption of a more or less smooth age-related increase in pathology, a reasonable presumption with respect to males. However, the exam procedure seldom changes on a premenopausal vs. postmenopausal basis. Women vaguely understand that "hot flashes," "jitteriness," etc., have something to do with hormonal changes. Attending physicians treat symptoms and prescribe hormonal therapy but do not always adequately educate women as to the fundamental physiologic changes implicit during menopause. Both examinations and education programs in industry are usually lacking in this respect.

Fourth, the logistics and atmosphere of periodic examination programs, whether in-house, clinic, or physician's office, are geared to the male patient. Open-back robes (or no robes at all) are acceptable to many males but repulsive to most women. Inadequate privacy in lavatory and dressing rooms, rolldown socks and shoes, clumsy techniques with an ice cold speculum, etc., reflect inadequate response to women's needs. At EHE's main clinic in New York, this issue was faced ten years ago. Questionnaires distributed to the female employees of a large client revealed substantial dissatisfaction in these areas. In response, EHE developed its "Woman's Day" program: regularly scheduled examination sessions during the workday and in the evening where all clinic facilities are closed to men. A female gynecologist is in attendance. Little touches such as wrap-around gowns, special slippers, and flowers were introduced. More importantly, an internal in-service training program for medical staff on the special needs of women is in progress. At present, appointment backlogs run two to three weeks for general examination sessions, but sometimes five to six weeks for "Woman's Day" sessions. As the proportion of female patients increases, the number of "Woman's Day" sessions will be increased as well.

Industrial periodic examination programs are generally limited to employees and most cover only "key" personnel. As a result, there is a huge disproportion of male employees being examined. And yet, a strong cost-benefit argument can be made for examining female spouses. The Health Insurance Association of America (HIAA) estimates that about 52 percent of health insurance claims are for dependents; of these, almost half (or 26 percent of all claims) can be assumed to be spouses' rather than childrens'. If periodic examinations and early diagnosis make sense for employees, then they make even more sense for wives. Since one-third of all hysterectomies are claimed by some to be unnecessary, the health education aspects of the periodic exam might also be effective in containing surgery costs.

A significant indicator of sexism can be found in a review of the forms that are typically used in the periodic examination process. Most often, the medical history questionnaire and/or physical examination record will have a section at the end marked "For Females Only." The questions contained in this section will frequently read along the following lines:

Are you pregnant?

Do you suffer from painful or irregular menstruation?

At what age did you begin to menstruate?

What is the interval between periods?

What is the duration of your periods?

When was your last period?

As we now live in a legally nondiscriminatory age, many of these forms now list these same questions under a heading such as "Gynecological," thus avoiding the charge of a discriminatory "For Females Only" approach. The result, however, is the same—primary stress on the reproductive system.

A brief examination of the changes women have recently undergone will illustrate the need for the health care field to catch up to its female clients. Within the past few decades, the American woman has been in a state of constant change. At one time, there was a widely held notion that women were generally divided into two categories: married women and working women. Only a few decades ago most women's lives were fairly predictable: the typical American woman married at an early age, had her first child soon after marriage, and had a number of children over a span of several years. A large proportion of her adult life was devoted to her family role of childbearer and childrearer.

Now, consider the changes. Today, in general, women are postponing marriage, postponing childbearing within marriage, and reducing family size. Add to that an increasing lifespan, and the result is a drastic reduction in the proportion of her life that a typical woman devotes to childbearing and childrearing.

The ability to plan births has made women more employable. Access to reasonably reliable contraceptive methods, plus an increased acceptance and expectation of paid work for women (who are now 43 percent of the work force), has reduced the birthrate and changed the timing of births and has allowed some women to be sexually active without pregnancy. Also, the increased divorce rate and the decline in the marriage rate mean that many women—some by choice and some by default—are leading economically self-sufficient and socially independent lives. All this change has brought about a tremendous amount of stress, and it is commonly accepted that increased stress makes one more vulnerable to disease. Today's woman does indeed need special attention.

We know that many women have accepted the primacy of "gynecology" as their principal differentiation factor from males. The annual or semiannual visit to the gynecologist is viewed by many women as a total annual check-up. On the other hand, an EHE survey clearly indicated primary concern in at least three other areas: nutrition, stress, and dermatology. These are discussed in greater detail below.

## Executive Health Examiners' Survey

Over a four-month period in 1978, EHE randomly questioned 161 women after each had completed her annual physical examination in our Executive Clinic in New York. The women ranged in age from 21 to 65 and 98 percent were employed, mostly in white collar jobs. This survey does not consider the more specialized needs of pregnant women, women working with hazardous substances, or women employed in what were traditionally men's blue collar jobs.

The survey participants were asked to rate certain proposed additional exam components, including nutrition counseling, dermatological counseling, and personal stress evaluation (psychological evaluation including biofeedback relaxation training). The responses were grouped into five age categories:

- *21–28: Early child-bearing years.* This group numbered twenty-seven, only one of whom had a child. The group favored the addition of a psychological stress evaluation to the annual physical examination, but rated the nutritional and dermatological components very highly. Only two of these women suggested components not listed on the survey: exercise and general health education.
- *29–39: Later child-bearing years.* This group of forty-eight women had a total of thirty-four children. These women clearly preferred nutritional counseling, followed by emotional stress counseling, then dermatology. The order of these priorities suggests that even though employed, their concern was still home-oriented.
- *40–49: Menopausal years.* This group of thirty-four women had a total of forty-eight children. A personal stress evaluation was the first choice for this group, seven of whom listed menopause as a topic of special interest. Nutrition ranked second and dermatology third.

*50–59: Preretirement years.* This group, forty-one women with a total of sixty children, preferred the nutritional component of the examination. This was followed by dermatology and stress.

*Over 60: Retirement years.* Eleven women over 60 years of age, only one of whom was still married, responded. The group preferred nutritional counseling, and rated dermatology and stress equal to each other.

It is difficult to trace a pattern in these preferences by age groups. There are, however, two clear messages: first, 97 percent of the participants agreed that the current annual examination format does not adequately cover the special needs of women; second, nutrition counseling was preferred overwhelmingly to the other suggested extras. As a result of this survey, EHE has developed a cost-effective nutrition program primarily to deal with overweight patients. The service will soon be offered as an option to both men and women.

## Special Exam Components for Women

The survey also showed us that more sensitivity is needed with regard to the whole issue of women and health. In designing a "Woman's Exam" at EHE, we elicited the opinions of many internists and consultant specialists concerning viable future programs. These examination components are geared to the whole woman, not simply to the woman as childbearer and childrearer. Although it would not be economically feasible to add each item every year to every woman's exam, our physicians and female patients agree that women need more information and professional guidance on fatal diseases, nutrition, dermatology, and various gynecological issues.

Diseases that kill, such as heart attack, stroke, and lung cancer, were until recently almost unheard of in the premenopausal female. But women's smoking and drinking have increased markedly, linked possibly to self-sufficiency and greater disposable income among working women. Stress-related illnesses are showing up more and more as women enter higher executive positions. Equality in the work force will mean that women will probably inherit the fatal diseases to which men have been prone for centuries. In the consultation portion of the preventive health examination, women will need to know more about their vulnerability to these diseases and will need a physician's help in implementing a preventive strategy. They will need to monitor their blood pressure more regularly than women of twenty years ago. They must be counseled about the other cardiac risk factors including obesity, lack of exercise, high cholesterol. There is overwhelming evidence to support the recent findings on the extremely high risk of heart attack and stroke in the woman who smokes while taking oral contraceptives.[2]

One out of every fifteen women in this country develops breast cancer. When caught at an early stage, this disease can be cured. Since over 75 percent of all lumps are first discovered by the woman herself, the consultation should stress the tremendous importance of breast self-examination, ideally on a monthly basis.

Women should be cautioned if their family histories include breast cancer. Such women should also be advised on the pros and cons of mammography. This diagnostic procedure must not be shunned solely on the basis of its theoretical risk. It is becoming more and more refined, requiring less exposure to radiation than ever. Although there is some theoretical risk involved, early diagnosis using mammography can be a life-saver in the long run.

Although the majority of women are abandoning the homemaker's role to accept outside work, housekeeping and food preparation continue to be "woman's work." In one generation, the role of the full-time housewife has become almost obsolete. With this enormous sociological change, we will see a shift in secondary schools away from the traditional home economics courses, and it will also become more difficult to learn basic nutrition from "Mother" since she too will be at the office.

Today, Americans spend one out of every three food dollars away from home. This figure is expected to rise to one out of two by the end of the 1980s. Concurrently, women and children are being bombarded by advertising extolling the virtues of fast food restaurants, snacks, ready-to-eat meals in a can ("just add boiling water and stir")—all with little or no emphasis on nutrition and caloric intake. Magazine recipes stress the beauty and glamour of elaborate food preparation, but often without regard to practicality, cost, and nutritional adequacy. Clearly, women need help supplementing this information.

Nutrition, as stressed by our survey results, is of concern to almost all women and increasingly to many men. This is where education, consultation, and a review of daily family habits could be of invaluable service.

A woman's nutritional program must be designed to meet her own personal needs (as determined easily through a history form) and tailored to her life-style, i.e., married, with children, working mother, etc. Obviously this consultation would not be needed annually. The basics should include some combination of the following:

Convenience foods: How nutritious are they? Are they all junk foods?

How to read labels: What to look for in buying canned or frozen foods.

How to eat in restaurants: What foods to choose or avoid.

How to prepare a quick meal with nutritional value. Are microwave ovens safe?

Food preparation for special cases such as pregnancy, illness in the family, young children.

How to deal with menstrual or menopausal cravings.

How drugs and foods interact; oral contraceptives and how they affect the diet.

Foods that are necessary to maintain ideal weight and good health.

This seems like a prodigious order, but a 30–50-minute consultation accompanied by written material could achieve all these goals.

A leading Manhattan dermatologist recently told us that many of his younger patients already anticipate and are saving for corrective cosmetic surgery in ten years. It is not our purpose to investigate or judge these trends, but this illustrates the fact that aging is now, probably more than ever, a major concern of many women. The women's movement may have a positive effect upon these attitudes, but it is still true that dermatological issues—acne, dry skin, cosmetic allergies, and facial hair—are more a woman's concern than a man's.

Some form of dermatological examination could easily be added to the current examination process. It could include advice on daily skin care, information on minor corrective measures (for moles, lesions, dilated blood vessels), make-up counseling based on what is good for the skin over the short and long term, and an outline of the pros and cons of face lifts when a person requests this information.

The current gynecological exam is sufficient for detecting certain "female" diseases, but this is one of the many health issues that should not be judged solely in terms of disease findings. Rather, the exam should be educational, informative, and instructive as well. The two most important elements of a gynecological exam are the physician's time and his or her willingness to carry on a dialog with the patient. Women are no longer satisfied with the paternalistic attitude many physicians assumed in the past. They want to be—and should be—full partners in the discussion of their health and the choice of treatment they face. There must be an openness to discuss difficult gynecological issues such as the risks of various birth control devices, vaginitis, venereal diseases (when they are uncovered), sterilization, failure to achieve orgasm, breast surgery, and menopause. A perfunctory examination of the female organs is not sufficient, in our experience, to deal with the many complex sexual issues and choices facing women.

## Recommendations

Women's attachment to the labor force is becoming more and more permanent, and women will expect the same benefits as men with similar work attachments. Because the growth of the economy is dependent upon having a sufficient supply of able workers and because women have been responding at an increasing rate to rising demands, promoting and conserving the health of women workers is essential. We must alter health care to meet women's needs and concerns.

The first step in this process is education. Women must be taught that an annual Pap test, pelvic, and breast examination is not sufficient. They need to understand the purpose of a complete diagnostic physical examination and be encouraged to demand it. Their need for such an examination is highlighted by the fact that women lose more workdays because of acute conditions, other than injuries, per employed person than men, according to the Health Insurance Institute.[3]

Medical practitioners, especially obstetricians and gynecologists, must be counseled to perform more complete examinations on their patients or to recommend that they seek such examinations from an internist, preventive health clinic, or family practitioner.

Industry, too, must be educated in the health needs of women workers. Industry must be guided to examine their current policies on health care and to identify discriminatory services. For instance, if participation in an annual examination program is determined by salary or grade level rather than age, women may be eliminated just by the mere fact that they have not yet made inroads to those levels.

Once women are brought into the preventive health care system, we must provide services that meet their specific needs. Given that the annual diagnostic physical examination provides a basic inventory of all bodily systems and a very good idea of general well-being, we can use it as a foundation for a total health survey for a woman.

---

**NOTES**
1. E.g., J. R. Willson, C. T. Beecham, and E. R. Carrington, *Obstetrics and Gynecology*, 4th ed. (St. Louis: Mosby, 1971).
2. P. Dillon and J. Seasholtz, "Oral Contraceptives and Myocardial Infarction," *Cardiovascular Nursing* 15 (March–April 1979): 5–9.
3. *Source Book of Health Insurance Data, 1977–1978* (Washington, D.C.: Health Insurance Institute).

# Appendix: Recommended Women's Examinations

We at EHE recommend the following basic examinations to meet the full range of needs and requirements of women in all age groups.

## Premenopausal

1. Medical history, annually.
2. Physical examination of all body systems (preferably by a female gynecologist), including a Pap smear, pelvic examination, breast examination, and instruction on breast self-examination.
3. Nutrition consultation, optional, or as recommended by physician.
4. Dermatology profile, optional, or as recommended by physician.
5. Psychological ("stress") evaluation, optional, or as recommended by physician.
6. Chest x-ray: smoker—annually; nonsmoker—once for baseline reference, then every three years unless pulmonary symptoms develop.
7. Electrocardiogram, once for baseline reference unless cardiac symptoms develop.
8. Pulmonary function: smoker—annually; nonsmoker—once for baseline reference, then repeat only if pulmonary symptoms develop or if patient is exposed to respiratory irritants.
9. Mammogram, once for baseline study between the ages of 40 and 45 for future comparison. (Various tissue patterns on mammography indicate higher risks of developing breast cancer in future. These patients should be followed more closely.)
10. Complete blood count, annually.
11. SMA 12, triglycerides, & FBS, once for baseline, then every three years unless increased frequency is warranted by medical history.
12. HDL-Cholesterol ratio, once for baseline; repeat only if indicates high risk of CHD.
13. Urinalysis, chemical and microscopic, annually.
14. Tonometry: under 40—only if indicated by family history or visual symptoms; over 40—every two years.
15. Audiometric screening: under 40—only if family history indicated deafness, frequent ear infections, or symptoms that warrant the exam; over 40—every three years unless symptoms occur.
16. Visual screening, once for a baseline record, then every three years.
17. Stool for occult blood, annually.
18. Proctosigmoidoscopy, once at age 40, then every two years if asymptomatic with a negative family history.

## Postmenopausal

1. Medical history, annually.
2. Physical examination of all body systems (preferably by a female gynecologist), including a Pap smear, pelvic examination, breast examination, and instruction on breast self-examination. The consultation should also include exercise guidelines for women over 50.
3. Nutrition consultation, optional, or as recommended by physician.
4. Psychological ("stress") evaluation, optional, or as recommended by physician.
5. Chest x-ray: smoker—annually; nonsmoker—every two years.
6. Electrocardiogram. Every two years unless symptomatic or abnormal ECG, then annually.
7. Pulmonary function: smoker—annually; nonsmoker—once for baseline reference,

then repeat only if pulmonary symptoms develop or if patient is exposed to respiratory irritants.
8. Mammogram, once for baseline study. Annually or biannually if strong family history (sister or mother).
9. Complete blood count, annually.
10. SMA 12, triglycerides, & FBS, every two years unless increased frequency is warranted by medical findings.
11. HDL-Cholesterol ratio, every two to three years.
12. Urinalysis, chemical and microscopic, annually.
13. Tonometry, every two years. Annually only if indicated by family history.
14. Audiometric screening, every two years.
15. Visual screening, every two years.
16. Stool for occult blood, annually.
17. Proctosigmoidoscopy, annually.
18. Cardiac stress evaluation, only if symptoms occur or if planning to begin a vigorous exercise program.

## Discussion

**Richard H. Egdahl:** What's the rationale for all of these examinations?

**Donna J. Morrison:** It's important to understand that most or many of the tests listed for our female examination are part of the general physical examinations given to both sexes. While it may seem like a whole battery of tests, only two or three items are designed specifically to meet the needs of women.

**Egdahl:** Isn't that discriminatory?

**Marcia Grymes:** It has been for years, I think. At least they're putting forth something for females. So few women are eligible for executive physical exams that companies haven't set up any criteria to use.

**Jeanne M. Stellman:** I wonder why nutritional counseling was uniquely a female concern?

**Stanley deLisser:** It was the service that women most wanted in our survey.

**Stellman:** But why isn't that also a male interest?

**deLisser:** It probably is except that women in society are more charged with food preparation responsibilities.

**Morrison:** We do have nutritional counseling available to all people taking examinations, including men, especially if there's a weight problem. But beyond weight reduction, many women feel that they need some help in knowing the differences between processed foods and so-called health foods, and what's a nutritious meal for their family that can be prepared inexpensively and quickly.

**Stellman:** The MR. FIT program, which is probably the largest clinical trial funded by the federal government, excludes women entirely which I find rather extraordinary. Yet that program includes nutrition education as an intervention technique. I really object to not including men in nutritional counseling because it perpetuates stereotypes and biases.

**William J. Bicknell:** I received two things today and noted some parallels between them. I got a new watch in the mail and I got the examination list for Executive Health Examiners. Looking at my watch, I thought it's very complex, extremely complete, very costly, clearly to me a mental health benefit, and clearly in the economic interest of the person who provided it to me. I wondered as I thought about that, without being too facetious, what are the benefits of this battery of tests? Have they really been thought through adequately? Something that is so exhaustive must be costly. Is this an accurate reflection of where we are in terms of looking at age-specific risk groups and targeted interventions? For these nonmedical, more behavioral concerns, how appropriate is a medical intervention or medically mediated intervention, whether done by a physician or nonphysician? I wonder also about the survey. How does one control the respondent's tendency to ask for more when the question is put "Wouldn't you like more on the exam?"

**deLisser:** If you want to look at the periodic examination as a case detection system or a case-finding system, you get into all sorts of arguments such as this. We are fortunate—we deal with a fairly narrow slice of the working population, basically the *Fortune* 500 companies, women executives, or wives of executives. I can only say we give our clients what they're looking for. The basic thing we sell is reassurance. People who come in want to know the state of their health and they can afford the expense. Secondarily, we provide health education and influence on life styles. We think these are worthwhile objectives.

# Sex Discrimination in Group Pensions

*John D. Blum, J.D.*

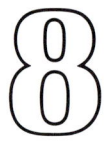

## 8

Recent judicial and regulatory developments have made it very clear that sex status alone cannot serve as a basis for treating women workers differently from their male counterparts. While rigid enforcement of sex discrimination laws on an individual basis is required, employers are often confused about whether civil rights laws allow them to make any distinctions between men and women on a group basis. A case in point concerns the ability of employers to differentiate between males and females in planning and administering employee pension retirement plans. This is an issue because, statistically, women as a group outlive men. The legal issue the mortality differential raises is whether an employer who treats women workers differently from their male counterparts for retirement plan purposes is guilty of sex discrimination. It is the purpose of this chapter to explore the legality of sex differentials in retirement plans as a vehicle for illustrating broader issues of workplace sex discrimination.*

## Overview of the Law

The areas of federal law that are most relevant to the topic of sex discrimination in the pension field are the Equal Pay Act,[1] Title VII of the 1964 Civil Rights Act, and the Fourteenth Amendment equal protection clause.

The federal Equal Pay Act, passed in 1963, requires that workers receive equal wages for equal work and that generally no distinctions are to be made between men and women for purposes of remuneration. Wage differentials are allowed under the act but only if they are based on a factor other than sex. The Equal Pay Act had been administered by the Wage and Hour Division of the Department of Labor. Under a recent presidential reorganization plan the Equal Pay Act is now administered by the Equal Employment Opportunity Commission (EEOC) as of July, 1979.[2]

Section 703 of Title VII of the Civil Rights Act of 1964[3] outlaws sex discrimination in employment; this Title applies to employers operating in interstate commerce who have fifteen or more employees. Fair employment practice procedures under Title VII are administered by the Equal Employment Opportunity Commission. While Title VII does not specifically address employer-provided retirement benefits, courts have been consistent in ruling that retirement benefits fall under the ambit of this Title. Under Title VII two possible defenses to a charge of sex discrimination are the Bona Fide Occupational Qualification (BFOQ)[4] and the Bennett Amendment.

The BFOQ exemption allows an employer to discriminate in hiring for a particular position or assignment where it is reasonably necessary for a business to have an employee of a particular sex; the EEOC has adopted a narrow view of this exemption.[5] The Fifth Circuit Court of Appeals in interpreting the word "necessary" in the BFOQ exemption viewed it as a business necessity and not as a business convenience.[6] Discrimination based on sex is valid only when the essence of the

---

*The purpose of a mortality table is to enable an insurer to calculate contribution rates. The table is not designed to show when an individual will die but rather to indicate a death rate of the group as a whole. The death rate determines the insurer's cost and the cost contribution level. A mortality table can be composed of various groups of individuals but the groupings need to be large enough to allow the law of averages to operate. Insurers favor groupings that include the largest number of similar individuals and that the similarity they share be one that is predictive of longevity. It is thus logical that sex would serve as a desirable grouping characteristic for insurers because it both groups a very large category of individuals and has proven highly predictive of individual longevity.

business operation would be undermined by not allowing the challenged practice.[7] By essence of the business practice is meant that which is necessary for the safe and efficient operation of a business.

The Bennett Amendment[8] to Title VII incorporates section 206(d) of the Equal Pay Act into that Title, allowing an employer to pay men and women different wages for the same job only if such differential is not based on sex. The legislative history of the Equal Pay Act indicates that wage differentials between the sexes would have to be based upon a specific and ascertainable additional cost for each employee. Whether on the basis of either the EEOC position or judicial interpretation, it does not seem that the Bennett Amendment's allowance of a wage differential applies in a situation where an employer bases the differential on the average cost of employing women as a group as opposed to the average cost of employing a group of men.

The equal protection clause of the Fourteenth Amendment guarantees every person equal treatment under law. To be consistent with the equal protection clause, individual or group classifications have to be reasonable and not arbitrary, resting on a fair and substantial relation to the object of the legislation (or regulation), so that all persons similarly situated are treated alike.[9] The test most often used to evaluate whether someone has been discriminated against under the Fourteenth Amendment is the rational basis test. If either a suspect classification (i.e., race, religion) or a fundamental interest is involved, courts will exercise strict scrutiny in evaluating the Fourteenth Amendment challenge.

Sex has not been regarded as a suspect classification but it has been placed in an intermediate category with a separate test applied to it. The U.S. Supreme Court has required that a classification based on sex "must serve important governmental objectives and must be substantially related to achievement of those objectives."[10] While not as severe a test as strict scrutiny, the sex classification test does not presume the questioned practice to be constitutional as in the case with the less stringent rational basis test.

## The Cases

### City of Los Angeles v. Manhart

In the case of *City of Los Angeles Department of Water and Power v. Manhart*,[11] the U.S. Supreme Court was faced with the issue of whether Title VII of the 1964 Civil Rights Act banned an employer from requiring female workers to make greater contributions to a pension retirement fund because of group mortality experience.

The facts leading up to this action were as follows. Marie Manhart was employed by the City of Los Angeles Department of Water and Power and participated in the employer pension plan. This was a defined benefit plan that provided equal monthly benefits upon retirement for men and women of the same age, seniority, and service. Benefits were funded entirely by contributions from the employees and the department, augmented by income earned on those contributions. No private insurance company was involved in the administration of payment of benefits. On the basis of mortality tables and its own experience, the department determined that its two thousand female employees would outlive the male employees by several years. Thus the cost of the pension plan was greater for the average retired female than for the average retired male. To offset the disparity in payouts the department required female employees to contribute 14.84 percent more of their monthly pay to the pension fund.

Ms. Manhart brought a class action suit in 1973 in the U.S. District Court for the Central District of California challenging the department's practice of setting contributions based on sex as a violation of Title VII.* The District Court in a motion for summary judgment ruled that the contribution requirement was violative of section 703(a)(1) and ordered a refund of all excess contributions; the decision was affirmed by the Ninth Circuit Court of Appeals.

In bringing the case before the U.S. Supreme Court, the department contended that the differential in take-home pay between men and women was not a violation of Title VII because (1) the difference in take-home pay was offset by the difference in pension benefits for men and women; (2) the differential was based on a factor other than sex within the meaning of the Equal Pay Act and was therefore protected by the Bennett Amendment; (3) the rationale of *General Electric Co. v. Gilbert* (492 U.S. 125) requires reversal; and (4) the retroactive monetary recovery is unjustified.

In considering the department's argument that class differences justified pension payment differentials, the court stated, "Practices which classify employees in terms of religion, race, or sex tend to preserve traditional assumptions about groups rather than thoughtful scrutiny of individuals." The practice in question hinged solely on the individuals' sex and as such constituted discrimination. The court rejected the department's contention that the retirement benefits of women workers, unless assessed an extra charge, would be subsidized by the male workers' contributions: "When insurance risks are

---

*While the *Manhart* case was pending in the District Court, California passed a law prohibiting certain municipal departments from requiring female workers to make higher pension fund contributions. The department amended its plan so that no distinctions were made in either contributions or benefits on the basis of sex.

grouped, the better risk always subsidizes the poorer risk. Healthy persons subsidize medical benefits for the less healthy . . . ; persons who eat, drink, or smoke to excess may subsidize pension benefits for persons whose habits are more temperate . . . nothing more than habit makes one subsidy seem less fair than the other."

The department contended that exception four to the Equal Pay Act was applicable in this situation, namely, that a payment differential between men and women could be justified if it was based on a factor other than sex. The department position was that the differences in contributions resulted from differences in longevity rather than sex. The court rejected the argument, noting that no evidence was presented that the 14.84 percent difference for female payments was based on any factor other than sex. The employer relied on a remark made by Senator Hubert Humphrey during the debate on the 1964 Civil Rights Act that this statute was not meant to affect the differences in treatment between the sexes in industrial benefit plans. The court, however, concluded that Senator Humphrey's statements could not outweigh the plain language of the Equal Pay Act.

The department argued that reversal was required on the basis of the *General Electric Co. v. Gilbert* case. In *Gilbert*, the court had ruled that an employer could exclude pregnancy from a disability plan without engaging in sex discrimination. The rationale behind the *Gilbert* decision was that the discrimination in question was not based upon sex but rather upon a physical condition. The court did not accept the department's argument that *Gilbert* mandated reversal, but distinguished that case from the one at bar: "The General Electric plan did not involve discrimination based upon gender as such. The two groups of potential recipients which the *Gilbert* case concerned were pregnant women and nonpregnant persons. While the first group is exclusively female, the second includes members of both sexes . . . . In contrast, each of the two groups of employees involved in this case is composed entirely and exclusively of members of the same sex. On its face, this plan discriminates on the basis of sex whereas the General Electric plan discriminated on the basis of a special physical disability."

The employer further argued that the absence of a discriminatory effect on women as a class justifies an employment practice that may discriminate against an individual. However, once it was established that prima facie discrimination existed, the court argued that the effect on class was meaningless. The court stated, "In essence the employer is arguing that the prima facie showing of discrimination based on evidence of different contributions for the respective sexes is rebutted by its demonstration that there is a like difference in the cost of providing benefits for the respective classes. That argument might prevail if Title VII contained a cost justification defense . . . . But neither Congress nor the courts have recognized such a defense under Title VII."

Last, the court considered the department's argument that in this situation retroactive monetary recovery is unjustifiable, a question of remedy rather than legal substantive. On this issue, the court agreed with the employer. Whether back pay is ordered under a Title VII challenge remains within judicial discretion, but there is a presumption in favor of doing so. The court felt that retroactive relief was inappropriate because of the conflict among governmental agencies on this point, the length of time it takes to amend a retirement plan, and the possibility of jeopardizing an insurer's solvency and thus an insured's benefits.

Viewed in a broad context, Manhart can be read to stand for the proposition that no sex differential affecting individuals in employee benefit plans will be tolerated under Title VII, even if the group characteristics are measurable and well-established. And yet the court states that the decision applies only to the situation at hand and is not designed to alter insurance industry practices in the pension field. This modification makes the interpretation of the case difficult, for while the opinion indicates that sex distinctions in the employee retirement area may be allowable, such a position does not seem to square with the face of the opinion.

## EEOC v. Colby College

While Manhart dealt with the question of discrimination in contribution requirements, the very recent case of EEOC v. Colby College[12] raised the issue of the legality of lower annuity payouts to female employees. In this situation Colby College provided faculty and staff with a retirement annuity through a contributory pension plan purchased from Teachers Insurance Annuity Association (TIAA); the college required that all eligible employees participate in the plan. Under this plan women employees received smaller monthly annuity payments than men with the same number of years of participation, age, and salary, even though all contributions were equal. The reason for the disparity resulted from the fact that TIAA, as is most common, determined the amount of coverage it would supply for a given premium by use of mortality tables segregated by sex.\* The Colby College women received smaller monthly annuities because as a group they lived longer than their male counterparts and hence received more payments.

\*Most private pension plans use the "defined benefits" approach in which benefits are calculated on the basis of years of service and compensation. In such plans actuarial tables are not used directly in setting individual benefits, although they are used in predicting cost. The other common form of private pension plans is the "defined contribution" plan in which contributions are made to the plan at a fixed rate for years of service and benefits are calculated on retirement as the amount that can be purchased with the accumulated contributions.

This action was brought by EEOC on the basis of a complaint made by a retired woman faculty member who alleged that she was being discriminated against under Title VII because of the disparity in annuity payments. The district court found that the actuarial value of the TIAA annuity contracts written on employees was the same regardless of the fact that the monthly payments were larger for men than women. The action was dismissed as not being a violation of Title VII but was viewed by the court as permissible under the Equal Pay Act.

The EEOC appealed the district court decision, relying heavily on the *Manhart* case which had since been decided. In relying on the *Manhart* opinion the Court of Appeals held that the receipt of smaller annuity payments by women faculty members was in violation of Title VII. "If the statute's focus on the individual forbids an employer from treating women as a class with respect to annuities so as to require from them higher premiums, although they as a class receive more for their money, it is difficult to perceive a distinction that would permit a plan whereby women make contributions equal to those of men but receive smaller monthly payments." The court rejected the position that in the case of employee insurance benefits Colby College was only an intermediary, but took the position that an employer's adoption of an insurance program (in this case, TIAA) made the employer an affirmative, active participant in the program. The fact that Colby made equal contributions on behalf of both sexes did not change the fact that women annuitants were discriminated against. The court noted that contributions were not made in the form of payment with which an employee could do as he/she desired; rather they could only be used to purchase an annuity that gave women less for their dollars than men.

In the *Colby College* case the court was very aware that the group discrimination issue raised serious questions about how employers must deal with pension plans so as not to be guilty of a Title VII violation. The court pointed out that the statistical discrepancy between male and female mortality is one that cannot be ignored by an insurance company. The law forbidding discrimination in this area leads an employer to two possible courses of action that result in payment of a supplement to the female work force. The first option would be for the employer to make up the difference between the male and female groups by paying an amount that would result in equal benefits to both groups. Such a solution would not follow *Manhart* which characterized the pension benefit as compensation under Title VII. Larger contributions on behalf of female workers by an employer is a form of discrimination and impermissible on its face.

The other possibility here would be for the insurers to devise a unisex table so that employer contributions for men and women are the same. Besides the fact that the insurance industry has never used unisex mortality tables, the court indicates that the use of one would raise a number of complex legal issues. In a unisex table male workers who live shorter periods of time would subsidize females; such a subsidy would be variable depending upon the male/female composition of pension plan participants and, according to the *Colby* court, "a variable subsidy would upset the widely desired practical definiteness in pension plans." A male subsidy may create contractual problems in plans where male contributions are already agreed upon; such a change in contribution may be challenged as a breach of contract. Where a female subsidy existed in a pension that allowed for a lump sum option, a woman's surrender value would be larger than a man's. If in a lump sum option plan the surrender values were equalized, the amount payable to men would be greater than the true actuarial value; men would thus be likely to opt for one-sum payment, leaving the pension plan with inadequate funds to cover a large female constituency. The *Colby* court did not provide answers to the problem areas it flagged but succeeded in demonstrating that the pension discrimination question, so intertwined with insurance practices, presented issues far more complex than those raised by *Manhart*.

## Reilly v. Robertson

In the Indiana case of *Reilly v. Robertson*,[13] a teachers' retirement fund appealed a lower court decision that found the fund's treatment of women annuitants in violation of federal law. Mary Robertson, a retired Indiana schoolteacher, challenged the Indiana Teachers' Retirement Fund practice of paying females $15 less per month than males of the same age and service. As in the *Colby College* case, the women teachers paid the same amount as men, but because of group discrepancies in life span drawn from mortality tables, women received smaller retirement payments.

Unlike the *Colby* case, the *Robertson* decision was based on a Fourteenth Amendment equal protection challenge to the fund's practice of differential annuity payment. At the lower court level it was decided that use of separate mortality tables deprived Mary Robertson and her fellow female teachers of equal protection and equal privileges in that there was no rational basis for the classification of retired teachers by sex. On appeal to the Indiana Supreme Court the state fund argued that classification of annuitants by sex promoted the objectives of the legislation by insuring the financial security of the fund. It was further argued that if men were required to subsidize the fund by receiving equal annuities, male teachers would be discouraged from remaining in that profession.

Basically, the Indiana Supreme Court adopted the findings of the lower court that sex is only one factor in life expectancy and others should not be ignored, that group mortality rates ignore individual experience, that experience shows 82.9 percent of females will have the same year of death as 82.9 percent of males, and that additional annuity income received by men will enable them to live more comfortably than women. In response to the specific arguments of the appellant, the court pointed out that there was no evidence that adoption of sex-based mortality tables would ensure financial security of the fund. The court was also not convinced that equalizing annuity payments would have any effect on a man's decision to leave a teaching position. Rather, the court stressed that a male teacher should recognize the fact that similar effort goes into teaching regardless of sex, and so would not expect more in retirement for his services than a woman colleague. The Indiana Supreme Court failed to find a sufficient governmental purpose in the teacher pension legislation that would justify the disparity of treatment between the sexes. The court stated, "the man and woman teacher when considered at the point at which each is first qualifying for retirement benefits, each of the same age, and each having qualified by the same number of years and level of service are not by reason of disparate group mortality experience dissimilarly circumstanced, and are entitled to participate equally in the right to receive payments from that fund made up of the contribution of teachers."

The fund sought to appeal the Indiana Supreme Court decision to the U.S. Supreme Court but was unsuccessful. The appeal based on a challenge to the finding of a denial of equal protection was not without merit. As mentioned, sex discrimination has never been raised to the level of a "suspect classification," but rather has been allowed when "it serves important governmental objectives and is substantially related to achievement of the objectives."[14] A reasonable argument could be made here that the goal of providing a solvent, self-sustaining annuity fund was an important governmental objective and that the use of sex-based mortality tables was a recognized insurance industry practice related to realizing the objective. The constitutional sex discrimination test was not used by the Indiana Supreme Court; it is plausible that if the U.S. Supreme Court had reviewed *Robertson* it may have found that the constitutional test was not violated.

## Conclusion

It seems clear that requiring women to pay more or receive less in a retirement plan because as a group they outlive men violates even the most recent Title VII tests. While there has been some debate, the EEOC position that sex cannot be used as the basis for higher contributions or smaller payouts in retirement plans is now the official government policy.* There is room for arguing that recognition of the sex differential in pension plans does not violate the Fourteenth Amendment equal protection clause, but such a position is only speculative.

Pension plans are designed to maintain postretirement living standards by replacing income. Strictly speaking, sex is not relevant to the issue of income maintenance; rather, the nature of employment, salary, and length of service should be of primary concern. Still, it is naive to think that sex can easily be ignored in retirement plans in view of the common insurance industry practice of using sex-based mortality tables. The courts have indicated that enforcement of discrimination laws is not intended to revolutionize the pension industry and have implied that sex differentials may in some instances be considered. The judiciary has not yet developed guidelines on how group sexual differences can be legally translated into calculating pension benefits. Until more definitive guidelines are developed, one is led to conclude that sex should not be used as a criterion in calculating either pension contributions or benefits. Perhaps a compromise can be reached so that group sex characteristics are figured into employee retirement plans without violating the law, but, in view of the current legal mandates in this area, it is unclear how that can be accomplished.

## NOTES

1. 29 USC §206(d)(1)(1970).
2. Presidential Reorganization Plan no. 1, 1978.
3. 42 USC §2000e–2(a)(1)(1970).
4. 42 USC §2000e–(e)(1970).

*Until recently there was a discrepancy between the EEOC and the Department of Labor's Wage and Hour Division position over the legality of having employers provide their employees with either equal benefits or equal contributions in pension plans. Labor interpreted the Equal Pay Act as allowing for either equal benefits or equal contributions; the rationale for the so-called "either-or" rule was based on an understanding that employers could sometimes purchase more benefits for men than women at a given price. (See Opinion Letter WH–70, Aug. 25, 1970 CCH–Wage Hour Admin. Ruling para. 30–681.) The Labor Department position did not account for the fact that because of the sex-based actuarial tables, the resulting benefits were larger for men than similarly situated women. On the other hand, the EEOC interpreted Title VII as prohibiting an employer from maintaining a pension or other benefit plan that differentiates in benefits on the basis of sex (see 29 CFR 1604.9(f)). After the EEOC position came out in 1972 the Department of Labor began a process of reevaluating its position in the area which culminated in August 1978 (spurred on by the *Manhart* decision) with the issuance of proposed rules that rejected the "either-or" approach (43 FR 38029). Labor's new position is based on the general premise that the Equal Pay Act mandates equal wages for equal work, and accordingly the department reasoned that pension benefits fall under the category of "wages" within the act. Further, Labor concluded that a sex-based actuarial table distinction is not a factor "other than sex" and cannot be used to justify a wage differential.

5. *Diaz v. Pan Am World Airways, Inc.* 442 F.2d 387 (1971).
6. Comment, "Title VII Employee Retirement Plans" 11 Loyola of Los Angeles Law Review 223 (1977).
7. *Robinson v. Lorillard Corp.* 444 F.2d 791 (1971).
8. 42 USC §2000e–2(h)(1970).
9. *F. S. Royster Guano Co. v. Virginia* 253 U.S. 412, 415 (1920).
10. *Craig v. Boren* 429 U.S. 190, 197 (1976).
11. 46 LW 4347 (1978).
12. U.S. Court of Appeals, 1st Circuit no. 78–1010.
13. 360 N.E.2d 171 (1977).
14. *Craig v. Boren* 429 U.S. 190, 197 (1976).
15. The Supreme Court case of *Teamsters v. Daniel* 47 LW 4135 (1979) deals with pension discrimination in general.

# Bibliography

Hankley, Thomas. "Title VII Employee Retirement Plans: Unequal Contribution Requirements as Constituting Unlawful Discrimination on the Basis of Sex." 11 Loyola of Los Angeles Law Review 223, 1977.

Hodges, Leo. "Do Equal Rights Mean Equal Contributions." *Pension World* 18 (Nov. 1978).

Huebner, S., and Black, K. Life Insurance, 5th ed. (Englewood Cliffs, N.J.: Prentice Hall, 1958).

Kaltenborn, Sara. *The Pension Game: The American Pension System from the Viewpoint of the Average Woman*, Report of the Task Force on Sex Discrimination. Civil Rights Division, U.S. Dept. of Justice, 1978.

Lavitzenheiser, Barbara. "Sex and Single Table: Equal Monthly Retirement Income for the Sexes?" *Employee Benefits Journal* 2 (Fall 1976).

Note, "Sex Discrimination and Sex-Based Mortality Tables." 53 Boston University Law Review 624, 1973.

Smith, Dianne. "Equal Protection, Title VII, and Sex-Based Mortality Tables." 13 Tulsa Law Journal 338, 1977.

# Discussion

**Robert E. Cooke:** We forget to look at the other end of the data when we talk about the greater absenteeism for women compared with men. If you want to compare loss of time in terms of economic impact, what about the problem of the much shorter life span of the male versus the female? I would think in the executive group, among the upwardly bound, that the economic loss when a productive executive dies at the age of 50 because of heart disease would have a greater impact than the year out, in toto, from a couple of pregnancies. I don't think that's been looked at by industry. There are enormous biological differences in terms of survival, heart disease, pulmonary disease. There are behavioral differences as well, although there is more drinking going among the females than there used to be. But I would guess that substantial differences remain as regards alcoholism in the work force between males and females. These tend to be lost sight of and only reproductive differences are emphasized. I think that's a bias which industry must reexamine.

**Robert M. Clyne:** Work was done at DuPont many years ago indicating that male executives have no higher incidence of stress-related disorders or heart disease than females. The differences appear in middle management and lower management and in the blue collar worker, not in the executive group.

**Cooke:** What I was speaking about is the statistical analysis comparing female and male longevity. You are going to have more deaths at age 55 in an executive group or any group if you've got 100 males than if you have 100 females.

**Stanley P. deLisser:** As one with a lot of years of selling industry on doing medical care programs on an economic basis, one of the problems of allowing for the cost of a man's dying younger by hiring women executives who live longer is that the actuaries are going to tell you about the cost of the pension plan which may offset anything you might save.

**Jeanne M. Stellman:** The last *Metropolitan Statistical Bulletin* has data on survival of women in the professions. Women when they enter into executive professions are not showing the increased mortality rates that some predicted. They are surviving the same way they survived in the other categories.

# REPRODUCTIVE POTENTIAL AND POSSIBLE OCCUPATIONAL HAZARDS

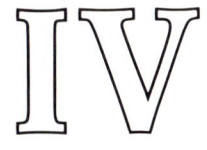

# IV

# A Legal Perspective on Workplace Reproductive Hazards

*Nina G. Stillman, J.D.*

## 9

By enacting such legislation as the Occupational Safety and Health Act of 1970 and the Toxic Substances Control Act of 1977, Congress has placed significant emphasis on toxins in the workplace and their effect on health. One of the problems industry must now face is the impact of occupational toxins on the reproductive systems of employees. This concern cannot be limited solely to females, since some agents affect the male directly and some affect the fetus through preconception effects on the father. However, with respect to teratogens (agents that affect the development of the fetus) and transplacental carcinogens, only the mother's exposure can be the vehicle for exposure of the fetus. Accordingly, the problem involved with exposure to

Portions of this paper have appeared in "Women in the Workplace: A Legal Perspective," *Journal of Occupational Medicine* 20 (September 1978): 605–609; and "The Law In Conflict: Accommodating Equal Employment and Occupational Health Obligations," *Journal of Occupational Medicine* 21 (September 1979): 599–606.

teratogenic and transplacental carcinogenic substances are sex-specific. Because the specific sex in question is female, legal questions of employment discrimination are raised whenever the employer takes action to prevent fetal exposure in the workplace.

## Preconception Exposure

Reproductive toxins can have a preconception and/or a postconception effect. A mutagenic substance is a preconception toxin that alters an adult's gametes in such a way as to produce a mutation in later offspring. If the employer discovers a mutagen in the workplace, his first inquiry should be, Does it affect males in the same or a comparable way as it affects females? The Equal Employment Opportunity Commission has indicated that any employment policy which prohibits or otherwise restricts the employment of women, but not men, because of the presence in the workplace of a mutagen that affects both sexes will be considered in violation of the sex discrimination prohibition of Title VII of the Civil Rights Act.

A second question the employer should raise if he suspects the presence of a mutagen affecting women in the workplace is, Can exposure be controlled in some way short of prohibiting women's employment entirely? For example, are there minor or practicable work assignment adjustments that will sufficiently protect the woman? Are there engineering controls available, such as improved ventilation or systems enclosures? Would the use of personal protective equipment, such as respiratory protective devices or protective clothing, provide sufficient protection?

Unfortunately, respirators cannot be worn by a substantial portion of the working population for both psychological and physiological reasons, such as heart problems, skin irritation, claustrophobia, and the like. OSHA's respirator expert who testified at hearings on vinyl chloride control, for example, has described all respirators as "instruments of torture."[1] My personal experience indicates that employees refuse to wear respirators, cannot wear them, or are constantly jimmying them for greater comfort. The problem of respirator acceptance is exacerbated when the substance involved does not give the exposed employee immediate physical discomfort, as is true of vinyl chloride monomer, an odorless, colorless, tasteless gas at room temperature and pressure. The employee has therefore no immediate incentive to keep wearing the excessively uncomfortable respirator. Protective clothing is similarly hot, bulky, and uncomfortable, and employees find that it impedes performance of their job duties. In fact, respirators and other personal protective equipment can themselves create hazards by impeding the employee's ability to see and move, especially in emergency situations.

Should an employer discover that it has a mutagen in the workplace, the spectre of legal liability arises from a variety of sources. Even if the substance is not expressly regulated by an OSHA standard, an employer may still be deemed to have violated the Occupational Safety and Health Act's general duty clause. An employee who has been injured by an occupational mutagen could seek recovery under a state workmen's compensation statute or other occupational illness statutes, such as the Illinois Occupational Diseases Act. Where a fetus or, ultimately, the child is injured as a result of a parent's exposure to an occupational mutagen, the employer may be subject to substantial liability in tort—that is, personal injury law suits. Under certain circumstances, the exposed employee may not be barred by workmen's compensation from bringing a tort action against the employer. We are beginning to see this in some of the asbestos-related cases.[2]

The issue of an employer's liability to a fetus or ultimately born child is as yet unclear. Nevertheless, certain trends in the law suggest that an employer may be liable to a fetus or ultimately born child who is damaged as a result of a parent's exposure to an occupational mutagen. One example of this trend is the decision of the Illinois Supreme Court in *Renslow v. Mennonite Hospital*,[3] where it was held that a child conceived nine years after its mother was negligently transfused with incompatible blood had a cause of action against, that is, a right to sue, the negligent hospital and doctor for injuries. The *Renslow* decision may have significance for employers. Should the court's holding be applicable to the employment context—and there is no legal reason why it should not—a child born damaged as a result of its mother's or even its father's exposure to an occupational mutagen will have a cause of action against the employer or former employer.

The application of *Renslow* to the employment context raises serious and complex medical, scientific, and legal questions. For example, one crucial element of proof in a negligence case is foreseeability—that is, whether the employer did foresee, could have foreseen, or should have foreseen that a particular act would result in harm. Here the role of company medical, industrial hygiene, and toxicology personnel becomes crucial. Anyone who suspects that the substance has or could have a mutagenic or other toxic effect must warn the company immediately. This is obvious and clearly falls within each group's professional code of ethics. But the more subtle problem is whether the company has an obligation in the first instance to determine whether a substance has any toxic effect before allowing an employee to be exposed. It is not inconceivable to me that in the not-too-distant future, a court will hold that in light of the ever-growing evidence of the toxic effects of occupational chemicals, an employer is obligated to determine such effects before allowing its employees to be exposed, and not just to control exposure after toxic effects come to light.

## Postconception Exposure

Concern with exposure of a developing fetus particularly involves teratogens and transplacental carcinogens. The problems are currently exemplified by the experience of the vinyl chloride monomer (VCM) and polyvinyl chloride (PVC) industries. In 1974 the medical director of B. F. Goodrich's Louisville PVC plant discovered that over the years, several of the PVC workers had died of a rare form of liver cancer called angiosarcoma. This was reported to OSHA and NIOSH in January 1974, and, almost concurrently, laboratory tests began to produce results indicating a causal relationship between VCM and cancer. Before the final VCM standard was promulgated, NIOSH made several recommendations to OSHA, including the following: "In view of the preliminary results of animal toxicology studies, it is recommended that no woman who is pregnant or who expects to become pregnant should be employed directly in vinyl chloride monomer operations."[4]

The bases for this recommendation were probably some early reports from Italy that exposing pregnant rats to VCM for only seven days caused their offspring to develop angiosarcoma, although the mothers of the offspring revealed no such tumors. From these experiments, it was concluded that VCM is a transplacental carcinogen and that fetuses are probably more susceptible to its effects than are adults. Yet despite the recommendation of NIOSH and corroborating testimony at the OSHA hearings by Dr. Irving Selikoff, OSHA made no reference whatsoever to VCM's transplacental carcinogenic properties when it promulgated the final standard.

Nevertheless, several PVC manufacturers have concluded on the basis of these and other studies that they are obligated to exclude women capable of becoming pregnant from jobs involving direct VCM exposure. The employers concluded that this policy was necessary because there does not now appear to be available any alternative policy or practice that will have a lesser discriminatory impact on women while still protecting the health of the fetus. The state of the technology is such that employers cannot control or guarantee against periodic VCM exposure in older PVC plants, and, for the reasons already given, employers cannot realistically keep women in respirators eight hours a day. Moreover, employers cannot merely transfer an employee after she is known to be pregnant, because an exposure could occur before the pregnancy is detected.

A fetus is even more susceptible to toxins than are adults because of its rapid cell turnover, immature biological barriers, relative lack of detoxification mechanisms, lack of drug metabolizing enzymes, and absence of a mature excretory system. One study with rodents, for example, has shown that immature tissues—late fetal or early neonatal—are fifty times more sensitive by dose to the transplacental carcinogen ethylnitrosourea than are adults.[5] The greater susceptibility of the fetus to a carcinogenic substance is also seen with diethylstilbesterol (DES). Although the mothers who took DES during their pregnancies have as yet manifested no significant abnormalities, the substance did cause vaginal adenosis in prenatally exposed young women.[6] Teratogens also demonstrate the greater susceptibility of the fetus to toxins; indeed, they may not even manifest a toxic effect on the mother, as in the case of thalidomide.

Both OSHA and the EEOC have recently given substantial attention to issues surrounding the exclusion of women capable of becoming pregnant from workplaces containing fetotoxins. Eleanor Holmes Norton, the chair of EEOC, has made several presentations on the subject to the National Advisory Committee on Occupational Safety and Health and on April 4, 1978, her agency issued a statement designed to put employers on notice that they may be violating Title VII of the Civil Rights Act when they exclude or remove individuals from the workplace because of alleged exposure to workplace hazards. Also in April 1978, Assistant Secretary of Labor for Occupational Safety and Health Eula Bingham sent a letter to corporate medical directors throughout the country urging them "to consider with great caution the adoption of any policies of exclusion as a means of dealing with occupational health concerns."

The issue of exclusionary rules has also surfaced recently as a result of EPA's decision to authorize the use of the pesticide ferriamicide, but to prohibit "females of childbearing age" from working with it. On January 30, 1979, Barbara Blum, acting administrator of EPA, sent a letter to Eula Bingham justifying the decision by EPA to exclude women. Ms. Blum agreed that there should be concern about sex-biased distinctions in regulatory decisions, but concluded nevertheless "that in some cases, such distinctions are justifiable." Ms. Blum's arguments were, first, that the toxicology data showed adverse effects in offspring of treated animals; second, that there was no way to provide protection for pregnant women, especially at the very early stages of pregnancy; and third, that employers cannot rely on the assurance of women that they are using an effective contraceptive. As Ms. Blum states, "How would an employer assure itself to avoid subsequent liability that the employee on birth control pills remembered to take them?" Additionally, Ms. Blum noted that routine pelvic examinations are impractical and probably "an unacceptable invasion of personal privacy." And finally she explained that a consensual waiver could not insulate the employer from liability for claims on behalf of the injured child.

Clearly, the problem of female employees working in environments that could have deleterious effects upon their reproductive capabilities is complex, pervasive, and emotionally charged. At this juncture, the conflicting objectives of different federal agencies as well as the dearth of relevant scientific and medical data have seriously hampered the development of a reasonable and consistent response to the problem which government, industry, organized labor, and the medical community can live with.

If the employer has a fetotoxin in its workplace, it should make every effort to determine, first, the effect of the particular toxic substance on the reproductive process and the fetus; second, whether the substance affects the reproductive capability of its male employees, female employees, or both; and third, whether the exposure which affects the reproductive process can be controlled or eliminated. Only if the medical and scientific data show that the mother's exposure could lead to fetal damage and that there is no way to control exposure should the woman be excluded from employment.

Thus, no woman of childbearing ability should be permitted to work in an environment where she could be exposed to a teratogen or transplacental carcinogen because only her exposure could lead to exposure of the fetus. By contrast, a mutagen may affect either the mother or the father. If the mutagenic effect can be carried by males, a policy that restricts only females will be held to be sexually discriminatory. Similarly, if a substance has both teratogenic and mutagenic properties, merely excluding women because of the teratogenic potential and ignoring the mutagenic effect upon males would be discriminatory.

The dearth of scientific and medical data relating to the mutagenic, teratogenic, and transplacental carcinogenic effects of substances currently prevalent in the workplace has created serious safety and health dilemmas for industry. If one suspects that a substance is toxic but the research demonstrating the effect is sparse, then to act on that suspicion to the detriment of female employment opportunities would probably result in a variety of legal and administrative agency challenges. However, not to act on the suspicion, but instead to wait until the data are sufficient if not conclusive, may be to wait too long. As a professor of pediatrics who acted as an expert witness in a case involving this problem in the vinyl chloride industry testified, she did not want to wait for ten, twenty, or thirty years to see if the two available animal studies were confirmed by the development of angiosarcoma in the children of female VCM and PVC workers.

## NOTES

1. Testimony of Edwin Hyatt, *Official Report of Proceedings before the Occupational Safety and Health Administration of the U.S. Department of Labor, in the Matter of Proposed Permanent Standard for Occupational Exposure to Vinyl Chloride,* June 25, 1974, p. 92/14.
2. See, e.g., Rudkin v. Johns-Manville Products Corp., C.A. no. 159524 (Superior Court of Calif., County Contra Costa).
3. 67 Ill.2d 348, 1977.
4. *NIOSH Recommendations for Medical Surveillance of Workers Exposed to Vinyl Chloride,* section H(viii), March 1974.
5. J. M. Rice, "An Overview of Transplacental Chemical Carcinogenesis," *Teratology* 8(1973): 113–126.
6. H. Ulfelder, "The Stilbesterol-Adenosis-Carcinoma Syndrome," *Cancer* 28 (1976): 426–431.

## Discussion

**Stanley P. deLisser:** Why is it that an individual can't waive the right to sue or in effect sign a hold harmless agreement with the company as the price for choosing certain jobs?

**Nina G. Stillman:** Cases on the subject say that you truly cannot inform a worker sufficiently and that workers do not have the right to waive their rights to protection under OSHA. It happens to be the law, rightly or wrongly—maybe we ought to change the law.

**deLisser:** That's what I'm suggesting. For national health insurance, Congress is perhaps going to say that a person who chooses a low-cost health insurance plan option waives the right to collect benefits under certain circumstances. Wouldn't changing this law be similar?

**Stillman:** First, I don't believe you can achieve this kind of result in Congress because there are too many trade-offs to get legislation passed. Second, situations frequently arise—for instance, in some of the states with informed consent for abortion or sterilization—where people say they were told but didn't fully understand the implications.

**Richard H. Egdahl:** In surgery and human subject investigation, our lawyers tell us that no matter how carefully informed consent is secured, no matter how much we explain, if something bad happens, it's a whole new ballgame.

**Jeanne M. Stellman:** Give me a male who works in a chemical factory, an aggressive lawyer, a deformed fetus, and a jury, and I'll show you a settlement for the fetus. It's a delusion to think that you're going to escape simply by getting rid of women.

**Stillman:** I disagree. It is much easier to present a case, to show that this woman had a fetus in her and that is the fetus that was injured, than to try to persuade a jury that the father's sperm cell was exposed to a mutagen. As a practical matter, it is going to be much harder to prove a case involving a male exposure at the state of knowledge we have today. If you believe a woman should have her choice, don't say that to employers. Say it to Congress so that some sort of law will be passed to insulate the employer from liability. Saying it to employers now is saying, Let her have her choice, knowing that the courts are ultimately going to hold you liable. In the real world, employers can let women choose only if they are given some protection, which they don't have at this point.

# The Biology of Toxic Effects on Reproductive Outcomes

*Jeanne M. Stellman, Ph.D.*

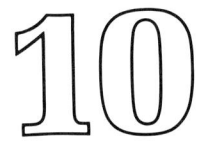

# 10

Perhaps 7 percent of all births in the United States are defective,[1] and an unknown but high number of pregnancies end in spontaneous abortion or stillbirth. In the vast majority of these cases—perhaps up to 70 percent[2]—the cause is not known. Hundreds of agents capable of producing such effects have been identified,[3] including many found in the workplace, but their actual impact on human reproduction has not been quantified.

Armed with the general knowledge that fetotoxic agents exist in the workplace, some employers now exclude all fertile women from jobs or industries where there is a possibility of exposure. Other employers, as well as regulatory agencies and public interest groups, have not yet established policy but are actively exploring the issue.

This paper discusses the scientific evidence implicating various agents encountered in the workplace as fetotoxins, and examines the adequacy of excluding fertile women *alone* as a means of eliminating the adverse impact of exposure. The case of inorganic lead serves to illustrate the points made.

## Kinds of Reproductive Dysfunction

Stillbirth, spontaneous abortion, and birth defects are three widely used measures of reproductive failure. These can be easily observed through appropriate studies. Other adverse effects, such as deviations from normal fertility and developmental defects in offspring that do not manifest for many years, are much more difficult to detect. All such outcomes must be considered when appraising the effects of working conditions on reproduction, however, and many may result from the exposure of toxic agents of either the female or the male.

**Organ Dysfunction**

Organ dysfunction, such as anovulation, implantation defects in the uterus, or the production of insufficient or defective sperm, may lead to infertility. Disturbances in menstrual cycle have been noted among several classes of female employees, such as women involved in the manufacture of diethylstilbesterol[4] and airline flight personnel.[5] Dibromochloropropane is one well-known male sterilant,[6] and many others have been identified.[7]

Unfortunately few quantitative data exist on the impact of industrial exposures on infertility. The dearth of information is not limited to toxicological aspects but extends to the basic mechanisms of infertility. In one report of 425 infertile males examined at a fertility clinic, a diagnosis of idiopathic causation was made for 25 percent—no etiologic agents could be identified.[8]

A major unanswered question is the effect of subfertility on reproductive outcome. We do not know whether the female or male who suffers sexual dysfunction but who is still capable of participating in the production of a viable fetus is more likely than others to produce a defective offspring.

There is some evidence that in males a selection among gametes for spermatogenesis occurs. As Manson and Simon note, mice have been found to have a high incidence of polyploid spermatogonia, an abnormality in the parent cell of primary spermatocytes. However, polyploidy among the spermatocytes themselves is rarely observed. Thus one can hypothesize that defective gametes or parent cells are selected against in the spermatogenesis process.

Defective sperm are present in the ejaculate of all species, and there is extensive evidence, both human and experimental, that sperm morphology can be affected by toxic exposure.[9] Unfortunately, the effectiveness of such abnormal sperm in fertilization is still not clear. Further, even if fertilization were to occur, the extent to which such defective fertilized ova could successfully implant and develop is also open to question.

Current evidence does not justify the assumption that natural selection processes preserve the human species from defective births arising from paternal origins. Studies demonstrate that mice do transmit chemically induced elevations in sperm abnormalities, and do so at the rate determined by Mendelian rules.[10] Manson and Simons discuss this more fully. Definitive epidemiological data on male factors and reproductive outcomes are not readily available, although suggestive preliminary work has been done on the effects of nonionizing radiation and some halocarbons.[11]

As with males, the impact of female subfertility induced by environmental agents on defective births is not known. Most studies have concerned the effects of exposure to toxic agents during gestation itself. Several other factors, like maternal age, have also been relatively widely explored. Maternal age, for example, is associated with an increased risk for Down's syndrome,[12] although whether this is due to normal aging or to environmental factors is not known. Animal experiments have found that organo-chlorine compounds can stimulate uterine growth and interfere with conception. It has been hypothesized that DDT exposures can cause resorption of an implanted conceptus because of DDT's estrogen-inducing properties.[13] The high miscarriage rate among operating room personnel exposed to trichloroethylene may be due to a similar mechanism.

Thus both sexes are subject to the effects of mutagenic agents and antifertility agents, and both sexes can become sexually dysfunctional. There is no convincing evidence to indicate that both sexes cannot transmit acquired defects to their offspring.

## Gestational Exposures

Even during gestation, it is apparently not the female alone who is at risk from toxic chemicals. There is evidence that toxic agents, such as the mutagen alpha-chlorohydrin and many others, can penetrate the blood-testis barrier and enter the testicular fluid.[14] Congenital defects, low birth weight, and poor survival in the offspring of male rabbits exposed to thalidomide have also been observed.[15]

Vulnerability to toxic agents during the latter periods of gestation can be assumed to be limited to the pregnant female, although she may be inadvertently exposed through contamination of the home by the spouse. The particular effects of industrial agents that act as gestational toxicants depend, usually, on the dose and also on the time at which the exposure occurs. It is not correct to assume that an agent will interact with the conceptus uniformly throughout the pregnancy. Generally, the fetus is most vulnerable during the first trimester when its organs and bodily structures are being formed. Also, it is incorrect to extrapolate levels of toxicant observed at one phase of pregnancy to other phases. Exposure levels during the first trimester need not correlate at all with levels observed in umbilical cord tissue, for example. This will be discussed more fully when some of the literature of the reproductive effects of lead is reviewed.

**Postpartum Exposures**

Birth has been termed more a landmark than an endpoint in the functional development process. The neonate, a wholly dependent and still developing human, can also be negatively affected by a variety of toxic agents via direct contact or through breast milk. It has even been hypothesized that the neonate may be more vulnerable than the fetus to some agents since it no longer enjoys the protection afforded by the uterine environment.[16] And, unfortunately, studies have documented contamination of the home environment with agents found in the industrial setting.[17]

## The Example of Inorganic Lead

Research on the effects of inorganic lead on reproduction provides illustrations of organ dysfunction, fetotoxicity, and postpartum toxicity. The following is not a complete review of the reproductive effects of inorganic lead, but rather a few examples of the various kinds of effects that toxic agents can induce. Inorganic lead is well researched in comparison with thousands of other agents in common use in the workplace, but even so, some of its possible effects and the mechanism by which it produces some of its known effects are still uncertain.

**Organ Dysfunction**

There is human and experimental evidence that both the male and female systems are adversely affected by lead but the data are inconclusive about its actual teratogenicity, i.e., its ability to cause structural birth defects. Several investigators have demonstrated that lead acetate fed to rats and mice can result in reproductive dysfunction, including abnormal spermatozoa with ultrastructural changes and hyperplasia of the prostate in the male and irregularity of the estrus cycle, fewer pregnancies, and an increased rate of embryo death after implantation in the female.[18]

In humans, Lancranjan et al.[19] have shown that men with lead poisoning, as well as with "moderate" and "slight" lead absorption, experience a decrease in fertility owing to disturbed spermatogenesis and teratospermia. The men also suffer disturbances in normal erection, ejaculation, and libido. Human and animal evidence regarding chromosomal aberrations induced by inorganic lead exposure is also available.[20]

Despite the evidence for chromosomal effects and teratospermia, the role of lead exposure in the production of birth defects in humans is not clear at all. In its review of the biological effects of lead, the National Academy of Sciences concluded that no adequate evidence is available which demonstrates this effect.[21] The reproductive effect of lead in animals appears to be decreasing fertility and increased embryo and fetal loss more than teratogenicity.[22] This appears to be true in humans as well, although definitive data are still not available and teratogenesis cannot be ruled out.

## Maternal-Fetal Transfers

Toxicological literature on lead provides us with data on its transfer from parent to the conceptus. It has already been noted that unwarranted generalizations about the relationship between maternal exposure levels and fetal exposure levels are often made. Inorganic lead is no exception.

Several studies of lead levels found in human umbilical cord blood and its relationship to maternal blood levels are available,[23] as are experimental investigations of placental transfer of inorganic lead.[24] It is clear that exposure of the mother to inorganic lead does result in exposure of the embryo and the fetus. However, the dynamics of the transfer are not clear. For example, Baltrop by examining fetal tissues, did not find evidence of transfer of lead in humans until the twelfth week of gestation,[25] and McClain and Becker showed that although significant quantities of lead are transferred to the rat fetus, the placenta appears to greatly limit the passage of lead because of large maternal-fetal gradients.[26]

These findings are similar to those observed for cadmium in rats.[27] Cadmium crosses the placenta at all gestational ages, but the dose absorbed by the fetus increases with increasing gestational age rather than as a function of dose. With cadmium a large maternal-fetal concentration gradient also exists. No available data, either experimental or human, provide us with insight into the quantitative relationship between the levels of lead and cadmium observed in the mother and those observed in the conceptus or offspring. The two blood levels are correlated but not predictive.

It is quite possible that lead may enter the early uterine environment via the semen, since the observation of polonium-210 in semen samples demonstrates indirectly the existence there of lead. (Polonium-210 is the radioactive decay product of lead-210, a radioisotope of lead.[28]) However, actual transfer of lead from the semen to the uterine environment has not been investigated or demonstrated.

**Postpartum Effects**

There is no need to discuss the adverse effects of lead on animal and human neonates since these have been extensively discussed elsewhere. It should be noted, however, several studies have demonstrated that lead workers have inadvertently exposed their families to this agent.

## Conclusion

This discussion has demonstrated that programs directed toward ameliorating risk to reproduction cannot be limited to females alone. At many stages of reproduction, both sexes appear to be at risk. It is possible that a given substance may affect only the female during gestation, but in order to establish this, one would have to rule out all chromosomal, spermatogenic, and other effects noted here. In addition, one would also have to demonstrate that the agent in question presented no general health hazard to the nonreproducing female or to the male.

---

**NOTES**

1. March of Dimes, *Facts* (New York: 1975).
2. James Wilson, in *Pathophysiology of Gestation*, ed. N. Assali, vol. 2 (New York: Academic Press, 1972).
3. J. Shepard, *Catalog of Teratogens* (Baltimore: Johns Hopkins Press 1973).
4. J. M. Harrington, G. F. Stein, R. O. Rivera, and A. V. Moales, "The Occupational Hazards of Formulating Oral Contraceptives: A Survey of Plant Employees," *Archives of Environmental Health* 33 (1978): 12.
5. F. S. Preston, S. C. Bateman, R. V. Short, and R. T. Wilkinson, "Effects of Flying and of Time Changes on Menstrual Cycle Length and on Performance in Airline Stewardesses," *Aerospace Medicine* 44 (1973): 438–443.

6. D. Whorton, R. M. Krauss, S. Marshall, and T. H. Milby, "Infertility in Male Pesticide Workers," *Lancet* 2 (1977): 1259–1261.
7. See J. Manson, and R. Simons, "Influence of Environmental Agents on Male Reproductive Failure," in *Work and the Health of Women*, ed. V. Hunt (Boca Raton, Fla.: CRC Press, 1979); and B. R. Strobino, J. Kline, and Z. Stein, "Chemical and Physical Exposure of Parents: Effects on Human Reproduction of Offspring," *Early Human Development* 1 (1978): 371.
8. S. H. Greenberg, L. F. Lipshultz, and A. J. Wein, "Experience with 425 Subfertile Male Patients," *Journal of Urology* 119 (April 1978): 1788.
9. A. J. Wyrobek, "Sperm Shape Abnormalities in the Mouse as an Indicator of Mutagenic Damage," in *The Testis in Normal and Infertile Men*, ed. P. Troen and H. R. Nankin (New York: Raven Press, 1977): 519–523; A. J. Wyrobek and W. R. Bruce, "Chemical Induction of Sperm Abnormalities in Mice," *Proceedings of the National Academy of Sciences* 72 (1975): 4425.
10. A. J. Wyrobek and W. R. Bruce, "The Induction of Sperm-Shape Abnormalities in Mice and Humans," in press.
11. P. Peacock et al., "Congenital Anomalies in Alabama," *Journal of the Medical Association of Alabama* (July 1971): 42: and Department of Health, Education, and Welfare, *Criteria Document for Trichloroethylene*, Washington, D.C., 1971.
12. A. M. Lilienfeld and C. H. Benesch, *Epidemiology of Mongolism* (Baltimore: Johns Hopkins Press, 1969).
13. H. C. Cecil, S. J. Harris, J. Bitman, and P. Renolds, "Estrogenic Effects and Liver Microsomal Enzyme Activity of Technical Methoxychlor and Technical 1, 1, 1–trichloro–2, 2–bis–(p-chlorophenyl) Ethane in Sheep," *Journal of Agricultural and Food Chemistry* 23 (1975): 401.
14. Manson and Simons, "Male Reproductive Failure"; and E. M Edwards, A. R. Jones, and G. M. Waites, "The Entry of a Chlorohydrin into Body fluids of Male Rats and its Effects upon the Incorporation of Glycerol into Lipids," *Journal of Reproduction and Fertility* 43 (1975): 225.
15. C. Lutwak-Mann, K. Schmid, and H. Keberle, "Thalidomide in Rabbit Semen," *Nature* 214 (1967): 1018.
16. J. C. Wilson, "The Current Status of Teratology," in *Handbook of Teratology*, ed. J. G. Wilson, vol. 1 (New York: Plenum Press, 1977): 47.
17. E. Baker et al., "Lead Poisoning in Children of Lead Workers," *New England Journal of Medicine* 296 (1977): 260; and Center for Disease Control, "Increased Lead Absorption in Children of Lead Workers," *Vermont Morbidity and Mortality Weekly Reports* 26 (1977): 8.
18. D. C. Hilderbrand, R. Der, W. T. Griffin, and M. S. Fahim, "Effect of Lead Acetate on Reproduction," *American Journal of Obstetrics and Gynecology* 115 (1973): 1058; J. R. Maisin, J. M. Jadin, M. Lambiet-Collier, et al., *Progress Report on Morphological Studies of the Toxic Effects of Lead on the Reproductive Organs and the Embryos*, contract ECE no. 080–74–4 Env. B., 1975; and P. Jacquet, A. Leonard, and G. B. Gerber, *Progress Report on Studies into the Toxic Action of Lead in Biochemistry of the Developing Brain and on Cytogenetics of Post Meiotic Germ Cells*, contract ECE no. 037–038/74–7 Env. B., 1975.
19. I. Lancranjan, H. Popescu, O. Gdasescu, I. Klepsch, and M. Serbanesci,

"Reproductive Ability of Workmen Occupationally Exposed to Lead," *Archives of Environmental Health* 30 (1975): 396–401.
20. G. Schwanitz, G. Lehnert, and E. Gebhart, "Chromosomal Injury Due to Occupational Lead Poisoning," *German Medical Monthly* 15 (1970): 738; A. Forni and G. C. Secchi, "Chromosome Changes in Preclinical and Clinical Lead Poisoning and Correlation with Biochemical Findings," in *Proceedings of the International Symposium Investigating the Health Aspects of Lead*, Amsterdam, Oct. 1972, CED, CID, EUR 5004 d-e-f, Luxembourg, 1973, pp. 473–482; and L. A. Muro and P. A. Goyer, "Chromosome Damage in Experimental Lead Poisoning," *Archives of Pathology* 87 (1969): 660–663.
21. National Academy of Sciences, *Lead: Airborne Lead in Perspective*, Washington, D. C., 1972.
22. V. H. Ferm and S. J. Carpenter, "Developmental Malformations Resulting from the Administration of Lead Salts," *Experimental and Molecular Pathology* 7 (1967): 208.
23. J. J. Gershanik, G. G. Brooks, and J. A. Little, "Blood Lead Values in Pregnant Women and Their Offspring," *American Journal of Obstetrics and Gynecology* 119 (1974): 508.
24. S. J. Carpenter, "Placental Permeability of Lead," *Environmental Health Perspectives* (May 1974): 129.
25. D. Baltrop, "Transfer of Lead to the Human Fetus," in *Mineral Metabolism in Pediatrics*, ed. D. Baltrop and W. L. Barland (Philadelphia: Davis, 1969): 135–151.
26. R. M. McClain and B. A. Becker, "Teratogenicity, Fetal Toxicity, and Placental Transfer of Lead Nitrate in rats," *Toxicology and Applied Pharmacology* 31 (1975): 72.
27. B. R. Sonawane, M. Nordberg, G. F. Nordberg, and G. W. Lucier, "Placental Transfer of Cadmium in Rats: Influence of Dose and Gestational Age," *Environmental Health Perspectives* 17 (1975): 139.
28. V. R. Hunt, "Polonium-210 Concentrations Measured in Human Semen," presented at 19th annual meeting of the Health Physics Society, Florida, 1973.

## Discussion

**Marcus B. Bond:** The lead case study is a timely one and it brings out some of the problems. We don't know that much about the effects of lead in spite of the fact that it has been around since Hippocrates or maybe even before. I am unsure myself whether I should let a female employee who is capable of becoming pregnant be exposed to environmental levels above the action level of 30 micrograms per cubic meter even if her blood level is below 40 micrograms per 100 grams of blood.

**Robert N. Clyne:** We know from Needleman's work in Boston, from Chisholm's work at Hopkins, and others' as well, that the fetus is very susceptible to lead. The Public Health Service has said that any blood level in a mother of higher than 30 micrograms poses a risk to the unborn child which may be manifest anywhere from two to five years following birth as a loss of cognitive powers and mentation. Meanwhile, OSHA's newly promulgated standards say it is okay for the first year to have 80 micrograms per 100 milliliters of blood, for the second year to have 70, and so on, until we get to 40 micrograms some five years hence. But that still doesn't protect the fetus. [See box.] As representatives of companies that use lead day in and day out, we must address ourselves to this problem. The only way we can do it is the way we have done it in Cyanamid.

I can assure you it has created more than just a slight murmur—an uproar would be closer to the truth. We concluded that we could not guarantee that the woman would have blood lead levels of less than 30 micrograms and so we had to exclude her—not because of any effect on her as an individual, but because of potential effects on the fetus. We worry about "loading of lead." Bob Kehoe, who has probably done as much work on lead as anybody, has made the statement that it takes twice as long to excrete a dose of lead as it took to accumulate it. There is a real possibility that a woman who works for two to three years in a high-lead atmosphere or a moderate-lead atmosphere and then decides to have a child some two or three years later after she has left the company may develop a malformed fetus or may abort as a result of the earlier exposure.

**Richard H. Egdahl:** If Cyanamid were to fix up the plant so that you would fall clearly below the level that would be dangerous to a fetus, do you have hard data as to what it would cost and what effect it would have on the price of the product?

**Clyne:** I don't have hard data. We looked at one plant in Willow Island that employs about 85 people, of whom 6 or 7 were fertile females. If we spent $385,000 on that one plant we wouldn't come close to 200 micrograms per cubic meter. A competitor of ours has just built a new plant within the last two years with all the existing technology and no holds barred as far as protective mechanisms are concerned, and they can't meet 200, much less 50, which is the OSHA standard.

**Egdahl:** You are saying it is virtually impossible economically.

**Clyne:** That's right: economically and technologically. The use of respiratory protective equipment might modify that statement somewhat.

**Bond:** There is another problem with lead. Although OSHA has said that the standard is 50 micrograms, we don't know that that is a safe level. The data on lead is human data from the turn of the century. The animal tests on lead have not indicated a safe level and theoretically the only safe level is zero. And you can't operate a plant at zero.

**Jeanne M. Stellman:** I find myself in an interesting position here. It

## WHITHER THE LEAD STANDARD

**1933** U.S. Public Health Service recommended 150 micrograms per cubic meter of air ($\mu g/m^3$) as a goal for industry in the 1940s.*

**1957** American Conference of Govermental Industrial Hygienists increased this recommendation to 200 $\mu g/m^3$.

**1971** American Conference of Governmental Industrial Hygienists lowered this recommendation back to 150 $\mu g/m^3$.

**1971** Lead exposure level set at 200 $\mu g/m^3$—based on the American National Standards Institute's recommendation—no reason was given for this level.

**1973** NIOSH submitted to the Secretary of Labor a document recommending lowering the standard for lead exposure to 150 $\mu g/m^3$.

**1975** OSHA proposed to the Secretary of Labor new occupational health and safety standards limiting exposure to lead to 100 $\mu g/m^3$ and recommended provisions for environmental monitoring, medical surveillance, employee training, and other protective measures.

**1977** Notice of hearings on the proposed standard was published along with an announcement of a proposed environmental impact statement to assess the effect of the proposed standards on the human environment.

**1978** Hearing record completed and certified in August 1978.

**1978** Standards for lead published in the *Federal Register*, November 14, 1978, with effective date set as February 1, 1979.† Standards contain requirements for (among others):

- Permissible exposure level (PEL): set at 50 $\mu g/m^3$—based on the opinion that to prevent impairment to the health and functional capacity of employees, exposure must be maintained below this level.
- Exposure monitoring: to identify sources and evaluate extent of exposure so that appropriate controls can be instituted and that employees know when they are overexposed.
- Compliance: employers must institute engineering controls and work practices according to specific implementation schedule to reduce employee exposure to lead below the PEL.
- Specific standards for respirators, protective clothing, housekeeping, and hygiene facilities.

**1979** U.S. Court of Appeals stayed the start-up date pending the outcome of petitions filed against the standards (January). The court then set the effective date for the standards as March 1, 1979, with limited exceptions.

Sources: *Federal Register*, November 14, 21, 1978; January 26, 1979; March 13, 1979; and April 6, 1979.

*Exposure levels are based on an 8-hour time-weighted average.

†The complete text of the lead standard is published in the *Federal Register* of November 14, 1978, along with arguments supporting it.

is always much easier to fight for lower standards than for higher standards but it is interesting to be in the position of asking why women and fetuses are being picked out for this kind of special protection? I have been pulling out all the literature on lead because it seems to be a substance that especially affects employee and personnel policies for women workers in industry. But it is not at all clear what the relationship is between a mother's exposure and the exposure of the embryo or the fetus or between the father's exposure and the potential effects on reproduction. Everybody cites a book by Baltrop [D. Baltrop, "Transfer of Lead to the Human Fetus," in *Mineral Metabolism in Pediatrics*, ed. D. Baltrop and W. L. Barland (Philadelphia: Davis, 1969): 135–151.] as the major source and he says that in the twelfth week of pregnancy lead finally enters the embryo. I looked up the original reference and found that the experimenter used fetal material from one mother and blood samples from another woman. The whole thing was invalid. If any worker actually has a choice about working with lead, my advice is don't because we really don't know what the effect may be. I resent very much applying the test of absolute safety and absolute security to the females as childbearers and not applying those same tests and criteria to other workers in our society.

**Clyne:** You are aware of the fact, of course, that lead has been used for many, many decades to induce abortion and that certainly occurred before twelve weeks?

**Stellman:** Yes, I've read that old data, and it is clear that there were toxic exposures for women. Women were suffering clinical effects of lead poisoning at the time it was used for abortions.

**Bruce W. Karrh:** You mention that the women were sick from the lead exposure. That is true, they were, but that study was never extrapolated far enough to find out at what level the mother was not sick and the fetus was stillborn. So we don't have a safe level of exposure, and we're right back where we started.

**Glen Wegner:** Lead is an appropriate item to discuss on a macro level as well because it illustrates the far-reaching economic implications of some of these health issues. There are only about twenty primary lead-zinc smelters in the country now, but I would guess that a significant number of them will have to close by the time they get the ultimate OSHA standards in place, if they do. The economic implications are mind-boggling, to say the least.

# Evaluation and Control of Embryofetotoxic Substances

Bruce W. Karrh, M.D.

# 11

The issue concerning embryofetotoxic chemicals is not that the female employee is more susceptible than males to adverse health effects from workplace exposures. Rather, it arises from substances that can cross the placenta and, at concentrations that would have no adverse effect on any adult, cause damage to the developing embryo or fetus. The female is involved only because it is she who carries the unborn child. Determining the potential risk from exposure of the mother to a chemical is a scientific endeavor, while deciding the acceptability of an estimated risk is a societal and regulatory responsibility.

Recent surveys indicate that up to 7.5 percent of all infants have developmental abnormalities that interfere with their survival or result in clinical disease. This is true despite the selective elimination of many malformed human ova, embryos, and fetuses by spontaneous abortion: over a third of all embryos die before recognition of pregnancy, and about 15 percent of recognized pregnancies abort spontaneously. Some estimate that about 40 percent of those lost embryos and fetuses would have been malformed had they survived.

Historically, lead has been used to bring on abortion, and at the turn of the century women working in lead industries were found to have decreased fertility and an increased abortion rate, along with symptoms of lead poisoning. This led to the widespread enactment at that time of labor codes forbidding the employment of women in industries where a lead hazard existed. In the 1950s Minamata disease was recognized and traced to the exposure of females to methyl mercury. At high doses, a woman becomes acutely ill and cannot become pregnant. At lower doses she may become pregnant but the child can be spontaneously aborted or born dead. At even lower doses, the child may be born with congenital Minamata disease, evidenced by neurological symptoms.

Maternal alcoholism is thought to be the leading known cause of birth deformities in humans, but the full extent of its effects is still uncertain. Of all birth defects, 20 percent are probably caused by known genetic transmission, 3–5 percent by chromosomal aberrations, and less than 1 percent by therapeutic and nuclear radiation. Another 3–5 percent come from maternal infections (rubella, syphilis, etc.) and maternal metabolic imbalances (diabetes, etc.). Drugs and environmental chemicals account for another 2–3 percent. The remaining 65–70 percent of cases are of unknown cause. This is the extent of current knowledge, even though the Thalidomide experience increased the determination to identify birth-defect-causing substances in advance.

The human embryo is most sensitive to defect-causing substances within the first month of pregnancy, a time when the woman usually does not yet know she is pregnant. Severe exposures during the first seventeen days after fertilization will usually kill the fertilized ovum, while sufficient doses between days 18 and 30 may well produce birth defects. Lower-level exposures to some substances for long periods may produce abnormalities that are not obvious at birth but appear months or years later. After day 60, the susceptibility of the fetus to agents causing structural defects decreases rapidly.

An embryofetotoxin is a chemical that affects the unborn child and may induce death, structural malformations, metabolic or physiological dysfunction, growth retardation, or psychological and behavioral alteration. These may manifest before or at birth or sometime afterward. The intrinsic potential of a chemical to be embryofetotoxic is relatively fixed. The response may be modified by the defense mechanisms of the mother and the target fetus.

Assessing the embryofetotoxic potential of the chemical (if known), the potential for human exposure, and the variability of the susceptible population provides the information necessary to estimate risk. An acceptable exposure level must be estimated taking into consideration the nature of the risk and one's confidence in the data. Then, potential exposures must be controlled to keep the risk down to acceptable levels. In deciding on control measures, the policymaker should consider the following questions:

1. Should employees at risk be informed of the possible consequences of exposure to hazardous substances?
2. Should safe-handling procedures be established and communicated?
3. Should engineering controls be used to the extent practical to reduce and maintain exposure to embryofetotoxins to acceptable levels?
4. Should such controls be augmented by administrative controls?
5. Should personal protective equipment be required whenever further engineering and administrative controls are not practical to keep exposures at or below acceptable levels?
6. How should employees who are required to use such equipment be trained?
7. Should women of reproductive potential be excluded from work areas where:
   - there is potential for exposure to an embryofetotoxin whose risk level is unknown?
   or
   - engineering and administrative controls and personal protective equipment are determined inadequate to ensure acceptable levels of exposure?

If an employer has considered each of these questions and the options they imply but still concludes that exclusion from the workplace (or administrative control of workplace assignments) of women of reproductive potential is the only feasible alternative, he must then carefully evaluate the legal considerations. Among these are:

1. Should research have been done to show that the embryofetotoxic effect is due to exposure of the fetus itself during gestation, not to preconception exposure of either parent?
2. Should research be done to show that exposure of male workers involves a comparable risk of damage to their children?
3. Should male workers be excluded from jobs where their exposure brings a similar risk to the fetus?

4. How should an employer's policy of exclusion be circumscribed to cover only those at risk? For example, in industrial situations where exposure levels within a plant and in nearby office facilities are similar, should exclusionary practices apply to both work areas?
5. While a practice of exclusion is in effect, should exceptions be made for any reason?

# Bibliography

Karrh, Bruce W. Testimony before the National Advisory Committee on Occupational Safety and Health. Washington, D.C., May 1978.

Done, A. K. "Perinatal Pharmacology." *Annual Review of Pharmacology* 6 (1966): 189–208.

Gibson, J. P., Staples, R. E., and Newberne, J. W. "Use of the Rabbit in Teratogenicity Studies." *Toxicology and Applied Pharmacology* 9 (1966): 398–408.

Health and Welfare Agency of Canada. *The Testing of Chemicals for Carcinogenicity, Mutagenicity and Teratogenicity.* (1973): 135–183.

Hurley, L. S. "Studies on Nutritional Factors in Mammalian Development." *Journal of Nutrition* 91 (1967): 27–38.

Hurley, L. S. "Approaches to the Study of Nutrition in Mammalian Development." *Federation Proceedings* 27 (1968): 193–198.

Jusko, W. J. "Pharmacodynamic Principles in Chemical Teratology: Dose-Effect Relationship." *Journal of Pharmacology and Experimental Therapeutics* 184 (1972): 469–480.

Kimmel, C. A., and Wilson, J. G. "Skeletal Deviations in Rats: Malformations or Variations?" *Teratology* 8 (1973): 309–316.

Koll, W. "Some Considerations Concerning Testing for Teratogenic Action." In *Proceedings of European Society for the Study of Drug Toxicity*, International Congress Series no. 73. (Amsterdam: 33 Apta Medical Foundation, 1963).

von Kreybig, T., and von Kreybig-Hackenberger, I. "The Basic Principles of Testing Teratogenic Effects." *Arzneimittle–Forsch.* 17 (1967): 390–392, (translation).

Murphy, M. L. "Factors Influencing Teratogenic Response to Drugs." *Teratology: Principles and Techniques*, ed J. G. Wilson and J. Warkany. (Chicago: University of Chicago Press, 1965): 145–184.

U.S. Department of Health, Education, and Welfare. "Reproduction, Teratology and Human Development." In *Human Health and the Environment: Some Research Needs.* (Washington, D.C.: DHEW, 1977): 315–328.

U.S. Environmental Protection Agency. "Guidelines for Registering Pesticides in the United States." *Federal Register* 40 (1975): 123.

U.S. National Academy of Sciences. "Environmental Chemicals as Potential Hazards to Reproduction." In *Principles for Evaluating Chemicals in the Environment.* (Washingtion, D.C.: USNAC, 1975): 156–197.

U.S. National Research Council. *Reproduction and Teratogenicity Tests, Part VII.* Washington, D.C.

Warkany, J. "Development of Experimental Mammalian Teratology." In *Teratology: Principles and Techniques,* ed. J. G. Wilson and J. Warkany. (Chicago: University of Chicago Press, 1965): 1–20.

Warkany, J. "Trends in Teratologic Research: Epilogue to the Third International Congress on Congenital Malformations." *Teratology* 3 (1970): 89–92.

Wilson, J. G. "Teratogenic Interaction of Chemical Agents in the Rat." *Journal of Pharmacology and Experimental Therapeutics* 144: (1964): 429–436.

Wilson, J. G. "Embryological Considerations in Teratology." In *Teratology: Principles and Techniques,* ed. J. G. Wilson and U. Warkany. (Chicago: Univ. of Chicago Press, 1965): 251–261.

Wilson, J. G. "Methods for Administering Agents and Detecting Malformations in Experimental Animals." In *Teratology: Principles and Techniques* ed. J. G. Wilson and J. Warkany. (Chicago: University of Chicago Press, 1965): 262–277.

Wilson, J. G. *Environment and Birth Defects.* (New York: Academic Press, 1973).

Wilson, J. G. "Present Status of Drugs as Teratogens in Man." *Teratology* (1973): 3–15.

Wilson, J. G. "Teratogenic Effects of Environmental Chemicals." *Federation Proceedings* 36 (1973): 1698–1703.

Wilson, J. G., and Warkany, J., Eds. *Teratology: Principles and Techniques.* (Chicago: University of Chicago Press, 1965).

World Health Organization. *Technical Report Series,* no. 364. Geneva, Switzerland, 1967.

## Discussion

**Jean G. French:** We must have some systematic way of letting people know what they are being exposed to. There are many chemicals today that we may feel are safe but which have not been adequately tested. Workers often have a multiplicity of exposures, and although they may not be in a position to judge toxicity, at least they should have the information on their exposures to convey to their personal physicians. We find that most occupational physicians are tuned in to what goes on in the workplace, but that private physicians normally don't even take an occupational history. Even if they did, workers couldn't give them an accurate accounting of the substances to which they've been exposed. Also, we've found that the workers in the dirtiest jobs are the most mobile, so they have toxic exposures in a succession of different workplaces. It becomes very difficult to piece together an adequate medical history to use in a diagnosis.

**Robert N. Clyne:** Of course you realize that the names of some of these compounds are literally a yard long and no way would the employee ever be able to present that to the physician.

**French:** What I am talking about is having a toxic exposure passport that would be kept up to date by employers, not information that the employee has to memorize and communicate verbally.

**Clyne:** Every process in American Cyanamid Company has a listing of all of the raw materials used for each final product. That is kept right in the department, and is available to an employee in the department any time either night or day. If you are talking about privileged information, proprietary information, since the companies have not been guaranteed by the government that it will remain proprietary and privileged, then I can very readily understand why they are reluctant to give the government information. When we get those guarantees, then there will be a different ball game.

**Robert E. Cooke:** As I understand Dr. French, this exposure record would be similar to an immunization record. I can't comment on the practicality of the suggestion, but I would point out that a few years ago in our textbook on pediatric nuclear medicine, [A. Everett James, Jr., Henry N. Wagner, Jr., and Robert E. Cooke, Eds., *Pediatric Nuclear Medicine* (Philadelphia: Saunders, 1974): 516.] we posited that a radiation record might be useful in regard to excessive exposure to radiation. The Food and Drug Administration is presently carrying out some studies on the feasibility of such records. It might be worthwhile for Dr. French to consult with her colleagues in the FDA to see how the technique is working out for following up excessive radiation exposure, largely in the medical field, with the aim to reduce mutagenic effects of radiation.

**Bruce W. Karrh:** The personal toxicity record would be good and we would like to see it except for a few minor details. But many employers have only one thing going for them—their trade secrets. Most employers have information available in the workplace which employees may have just by asking. They certainly have a right to know what they are exposed to. But when you start letting them carry that information around, you run the risk that should they become disgruntled over something they could go to the nearest competitor and hand over these exposure records, and it doesn't take a competitor very long to put together exactly what the company is using in its process. When the company loses its trade secrets it has lost its business. All employees have a right to know what they are exposed to and what the toxic hazard is—that was the subject of a discussion we had here a couple of years ago at a meeting exactly like this one. [Published in *Health Services and Health Hazards: The Employee's Need to Know*

(New York: Springer-Verlag, 1978).] But the problem gets to be how widely do you disseminate that information and who has access to it.

**Cooke:** One reason for letting the worker know is to aid in decision making, and the suggestion has been made that decisions can be left to the mother. I think the general population can handle the concept of probability rather poorly. That was found some time ago in the genetic counseling field, where the notion of probability really didn't make much sense to most people.

**Jean F. Duff:** Dr. Cooke's observation about public understanding of probabilities touches home because the group I'm with in Washington has been working on ways to display information specifically relating to health risk estimation for the general public. I believe we've much to learn about effective ways of disseminating rather technical information to consumers. We should try to preserve for the individual the option to assess risks. I think that the alternative of total regulation and total protection is not something that goes well with the sanity of society.

**Jeanne M. Stellman:** We "experts" may face that difficulty with probabilities even more starkly than the people we intend to protect. None of us knows what the probabilities are. We all make assumptions about probabilities that could be right or wrong and try to find some way to make the probabilities be zero or very close. We set our standards near zero and remove people in an effort to make our probabilities very, very low. We're not processing the probabilities that well ourselves, which may perhaps explain why it's so hard for us to transmit those probabilities to other people.

Also, economics plays a role, in that fairly simple and not very costly solutions are preferred. If it's very expensive to engineer the workplace down to a level that we think is safe, then we look for a somewhat less expensive option, which is to try to remove from the workplace the workers we think are at risk. Employers allow themselves choices among perhaps difficult options based on what's optimal for them, but the women aren't given the same latitude to face equally difficult decisions about where they're going to work and when they're going to stop working. We make the decisions for people. I believe that women can make decent choices, and that the essence of a free society is informed individuals making choices. If we're so worried about fetuses, what about saccharine? The animal evidence says that the second generation gets it. If we want to continue this protection of women and fetuses to the hilt, then should we not make it illegal ever to sell saccharine to women who are fertile and might become pregnant?

**Kenneth Edelin:** No, but I agree that the data on which we are operating are not that hard. One could draw up a very small list of chemicals and drugs and environmental things that we *know* will cause abnormalities in fetal development. At least 15 percent of all pregnancies end in spontaneous abortions. With the advent of sophisticated pregnancy testing as early as seven to ten days after conception, we know that some of those early pregnancies are lost, so it could be as high as 20 to 25 percent. When we consider also that there is a given percentage (maybe 5 to 10 percent) of congenital abnormality that we humans are born with, I wonder what the answer is. I don't see how the government can come out with the answers. That frightens me even more than a jury trial, quite frankly, and I've had some experience with jury trials. It seems to me that we have to recognize that we're not going to be able to reduce risk to zero. We see in the *Physician's Desk Reference* all the time the warning that "the safety of this drug in pregnancy has not been established." I believe women will be motivated to make the appropriate decisions. Our experience with fetal alcohol syndrome bears this out: 9 percent of our patients are heavy drinkers and the fact that they are pregnant is enough motivation to get them to stop drinking during their pregnancies. I believe that motivation can be used in industrial instances. We should talk a bit more about freedom of choice, because with the proper knowledge I think women will decide responsibly.

# Fetotoxicity and Fertile Female Employees

Robert M. Clyne, M.D.

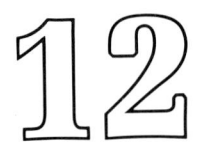

## 12

Two-fifths of those employed in the United States today are females over the age of 20, and almost 2 million more women are entering the work force every year. Women at work today number 42.8 million, compared with only 18 million in 1950. By 1990 they are expected to number 54 million. The majority of working women are of childbearing age—between 16 and 50. These fertile female employees carry approximately 1 million prenatal infants in American workplaces each year, according to Dr. Hunt of Penn State University. I must emphasize that this discussion is limited to fetotoxic agents; women are considered only because they carry the unborn children who are at risk of exposure. Effects on male reproduction are not covered here for this reason.

No single issue facing American industry today is as emotionally charged and controversial as protecting the unborn child from potentially toxic exposures in the workplace. The problems stemming from the rights of pregnant women to continue working until term, or from the recent legislation that defines pregnancy as a disability, are dwarfed by the dilemmas inherent in attempting to protect their unborn children.

## Government Disarray

One indication of the controversy is that government agencies cannot agree on what they consider fair and equitable treatment of fertile female employees. In June 1976 Dr. John Finklea of NIOSH promised guidelines on the subject in the very near future, but today, some three years later, none have yet been issued. We hear rumors that OSHA plans to address itself to this problem, but so far as I know they are still rumors. EEOC chairperson Eleanor Holmes Norton has observed that company policies on reproductive risk have "erred" on the side of caution and called for action to prevent discriminatory exclusion of women from certain jobs because of alleged hazards to their health. But Ms. Norton has erred in that the protective policies are concerned with effects on the *fetus,* not with effects on women, since women in the workplace are already adequately protected by existing standards. As a further indication of the emotion and controversy the issue engenders, Dr. Eula Bingham, the assistant secretary of labor for occupational safety and health recently exhorted physicians not to let discrimination against women occur, a follow-up to her prior letter to all medical directors in the United States indicating her concern about discrimination against women of childbearing capability who may be exposed to workplace hazards. Frankly, we were surprised that Dr. Bingham's theme was discrimination since her agency's mandate and priority are the protection of health and safety. Earlier this year, Barbara Blum of EPA indicated that fertile women should not be allowed to work with the pesticide ferriamicide which contains the fetotoxic agent Mirex. Dr. Bingham took issue with Ms. Blum, not on the dangers of such exposure, but on the discriminatory implications of the statement. Clearly, there is profound confusion in the very agencies that are charged with giving guidance to industry on compliance with their various standards and regulations.

## Kinds of Fetotoxic Effects

Recent surveys indicate that 4–7.5 percent of all infants delivered have serious developmental abnormalities. Approximately 14 percent of newborn deaths are due to congenital diseases, the third most common cause of death in this group. Further, it has been estimated that 15 percent of pregnancies terminate in miscarriages or, as the medical profession prefers, in spontaneous abortions. Undoubtedly this figure is low because many miscarriages are not recognized as such: they may be regarded as a delayed or late menstrual period by a woman who never realized that she was pregnant. Selective elimination of malformed ova, embryos, and fetuses occurs either soon after conception (between day 2 and day 17) or by spontaneous abortion of the fetus before the twenty-second week of gestation.

The response of the developing human organism to toxic agents depends upon its age. The first trimester of pregnancy is an especially sensitive time. Severe insults during the first seventeen days will usually result in the death of the fertilized ovum followed by spontaneous abortion. From day 18 to day 60, agents may interfere with the formation of the organs or other body structures, as thalidomide did. Because there is no reliable method to ascertain human pregnancy prior to three weeks after conception, a woman cannot realize that she is pregnant early enough to prevent fetal damage. The simplistic approach of removing women from a workplace after they know they are pregnant is not sufficient to protect their offspring.

The danger of structural defects is largely past by the second trimester of pregnancy, but other dangers remain. This trimester is a time of rapid fetal growth when placental bloodflow reaches its maximum level. In consequence, the delivery of substances to which the mother has been exposed across the placental barrier to the fetus can be enormous. In the last trimester, we have evidence that agents continue to cross the placenta and can modify the functions of specific organs in the infant.

A fourth time with special hazards is the immediate prepartum period. The mother's body may have been able to detoxify certain agents on behalf of the fetus in utero, but this protection ends with birth. If prenatal exposure has been extensive, the infant may be born with the agent in its tissues but lacks the enzymes or other metabolic mechanisms needed to detoxify it. Accordingly, a substance that does not appear to harm the fetus in utero may well be toxic to the newborn infant. Nor does the danger end here. Some fetotoxins may not manifest their effects until years after birth. Prenatal exposure to lead, for example, may bring on learning defects that do not manifest until the child is several years old.

## Kinds of Fetotoxic Agents

Toxic agents in our environment are not the sole cause of miscarriages or defective children. Despite the increased number and volume of agricultural chemicals, industrial chemicals, food additives, drugs, and other substances introduced into our environment, there is no evidence that human birth defects have increased in recent years. However, we simply do not know about why these unfortunate incidents occur in 65–70 percent of cases. We do know that 20 percent of all defects are caused by genetic transmission and 3–5 percent by chromosomal abnormalities. Radiation, infections such as German measles and syphilis, maternal diabetes, and other maternal metabolic imbalances account for an additional 5–6 percent of cases. Maternal alcoholism is the leading known cause of birth defects.

That some chemical substances have the potential to cause damage to a developing embryo has been recognized for a long time. In 1890 women in the lead pottery industry were found to have decreased fertility and an increased abortion rate. This led to the widespread enactment in the early 1900s of labor codes forbidding the employment of women in industries where they could be exposed to lead.

Another fetotoxic substance is mercury, identified as the cause of Minamata disease in 1959. This neurological disease was detected in Japan when people ate fish and shellfish from Minamata Bay which was contaminated with methyl mercury. If a woman's intake was great enough, she would become acutely ill and would not become pregnant. With a lesser intake she could become pregnant but the child would be born dead or aborted spontaneously. Finally, if a still lesser dosage were ingested, a child would be born with the characteristic signs and symptoms of neurological disease caused by mercury.

Perhaps the most dramatic incident of all was the thalidomide tragedy. Thalidomide is a tranquilizer that was used in Europe for several years. It was subsequently proven to be the cause of serious malformations of children when taken by pregnant women. The thalidomide experience did more than any other event to highlight concern about toxic agents and their potential effects on unborn children.

The foregoing are merely three examples of chemicals known to have fetotoxic effects. Many, many other compounds have been demonstrated to have similar effects, either in humans or in laboratory animals. Further, still other substances are highly suspect because their chemical structure resembles known fetotoxins or because of their other pharmacological or metabolic effects. The following is a general classification of agents which are reported to have caused structural deformities in fetuses:

Analgesics and antipyretics
Anesthetics, anticonvulsants, muscle relaxants, and stimulants
Antihypertensive agents

Antimicrobial and antiparasitic agents
Antinauseants, antihistamines, and phenothiazines
Caffeine and other xanthine derivatives
Cough medicines
Diuretics and drugs taken for cardiovascular disorders
Drugs affecting the autonomic nervous system
Drugs taken for gastrointestinal disturbances
Hormones, hormone antagonists, and contraceptives
Immunizing agents
Inorganic compounds and some vitamins
Sedatives, tranquilizers, and antidepressants

The known or suspected fetotoxic agents which specially concern the industrial medical profession are:

| | |
|---|---|
| Alcohol | Manganese |
| Alkylating agents | Methyl mercury |
| Aniline | Nickel |
| Captan | Nicotine |
| Dimethyl acetamide | Nitrates, nitrites, and other causes of methemoglobinemia |
| Dimethyl formamide | |
| Dimethyl sulfoxide | Nitrobenzene |
| Formamide | Phenol |
| Hexachlorobutadiene | Phosphorus |
| Hexafluoroacetone | Tetramethylthiourea |
| Hydrogen sulfide and other causes of sulfhemoglobinemia | Tris |
| | Turpentine |

Other agents that should cause concern in the industrial setting are three physical hazards: elevated carbon dioxide, elevated temperatures, and microwaves.

A third listing of chemical agents, called "Agents With Reproductive Effects," was developed by NIOSH:

| | |
|---|---|
| Aldrin | Anthrax |
| Alkyl Mercury | Anticoagulants |
| Amines | Arsenic |
| Ammonia | Asbestos |
| Anesthetics | Benzene |

Beryllium
Cadmium
Carbon disulfide
Carbon monoxide
Carbon tetrachloride
Chloroform
Chlorophenoxyacetic acids (Tri-, Di-)
Chromic acid
Chromium
Dyphenylhydantoin
Dichlorvos
Diethylstilbestrol
Diphenyl
Ethylene dichloride
Fluorides
Formaldehyde
Hair dyes
Halothane
Hydrogen fluoride
Isopropyl alcohol
Lead
Mercury
Methoxyflurane
Methyl alcohol
Methylene chloride
Methyl mercury
Nitrous oxide
Pesticides
Phosgene
Phthalate esters
Polychlorinated biphenyls
Radium
Selenium
Socium hydroxide
Styrene
Styrene oxide
Sulfur dioxide
Sulfuric acid
Thalidomide
Thallium
Toluene
Toluene diisocyanate
Trichloroethylene
Trinitrotoluene
Vinyl chloride
Warfarin
X-radiation
Xylene
Zinc oxide

Finally, NIOSH has recently developed a 2-inch thick listing of agents that can cause birth defects. Thus, we are not dealing with only a few substances—there are hundreds of potentially dangerous agents to which women of childbearing capability, but more importantly, their fetuses, may be exposed in the workplace.

## Protective Policies in the Workplace

The employer who has acted responsibly by trying to provide a safe and healthful workplace for the potential offspring of his fertile female employees has opened Pandora's box. When it has been established that a compound poses a risk of fetotoxicity, the employer should take the following actions:

- Employees should be informed of the possible consequences of exposure and appropriate safe-handling procedures should be established and communicated to them.
- Engineering controls should be used to the extent practical to reduce exposure to a fetotoxin to acceptable levels. Such controls should be augmented by administrative controls as appropriate and feasible.
- Whenever engineering and administrative controls are not effective in keeping exposure at or below acceptable levels, or are not economically feasible, personal protective equipment, where appropriate and practical, should be provided to and required to be used by potentially affected employees. Further, adequate training for the proper use of the equipment should be provided.
- Whenever engineering controls, administrative controls, or personal protective equipment are not effective in guaranteeing acceptable levels of exposure, or if an acceptable exposure level cannot be set, then females of childbearing capability should be excluded from affected work areas. Personnel managers, industrial relations and equal employment specialists, and medical personnel should address jointly the resulting problems of union contracts, transferring the employees, rate retention, and so on.

Allow me to emphasize once again that I am not advocating discrimination against a female employee because she is female or even claiming that female employees are more susceptible than males. The issue here is the fetus and its potential for injury through exposure to concentrations of a compound that do not have significant effects on male or female adults. The female is involved only because she happens to be the one who carries the unborn child.

It is important to consider one other facet of this most complex problem. On many occasions government agencies and union representatives have claimed that there is really no problem at all. What has to be done is to reduce the ambient concentrations of these compounds in the workplace to levels low enough to protect everyone: the male, the female, and the fetus. Oh, if that were only possible! But real-world technology is not that advanced. Even if it were, the costs of implementing the engineering programs would be staggering. Let us not forget that, with the exception of rare instances dictated by social needs, such as the manufacture of an unusual drug or strategically important compound, American business must make a profit in order for it and our country to survive. We must consider cost-benefit ratios as well as social needs.

Let us consider what may happen to an employer who, after weighing every part of the problem, decides to implement a program of restricting or excluding fertile females from working with certain chemicals. He may be faced with a grievance alleging violation of the terms of a collective bargaining agreement involving seniority or discrimination provisions. He may be subjected to charges of discrimination under Title VII of the Civil Rights Act. The EEOC has been meeting with officials of OSHA on such programs, and he may thus be subjected to intensive and prolonged OSHA inspections. It has been said that the EEOC will not bother an employer if the agency is convinced that the employee or the fetus would really be endangered on the job in question and the employer has made every attempt to transfer the employee but could not find a job to match her qualifications. NIOSH may decide to conduct epidemiological studies at his operating locations. The Office of Federal Contract Compliance Programs, the federal agency responsible for enforcing the nondiscriminatory restrictions on government contracts, may initiate a compliance investigation. If this agency decides that the company's policy is sexually discriminatory, the employer may be debarred from all government contracts. In addition, the National Workers Compensation Act introduced by Senators Williams and Javits and the Toxic Substances Control Act which is being administered by the EPA may also appear in this scenario.

There are compelling reasons why responsible employers must act and act now—not precipitously but in a reasoned manner. OSHA standards do not currently address the problem of the susceptible fetus in a meaningful way. But we must be concerned about the health and well-being of such a fetus. It has been stated that a mother cannot legally waive the right of her fetus or child to sue for damages, although this concept has not as yet been accepted by all. The consequences of a personal injury action versus a discrimination action must be carefully weighed and considered. The adverse publicity arising from a personal injury lawsuit involving an injured child can be far more devastating for a company than publicity about an employee discrimination action.

## The Decision-Making Problem

To conclude, I would like to record an actual situation that many of us have had to face in the recent past. In 1970 an epidemiological study indicated that the daughters of women who had taken diethylstilbestrol (DES) during their pregnancy to ward off a miscarriage suffered from certain vaginal abnormalities, including cancer. Naturally, all women who had used DES during their pregnancies were concerned about their daughters. Steps were promptly taken to prevent the use of DES in threatened abortions and the exposure of fertile women to this compound in the workplace. Now, close to nine years later, additional studies indicate that there may be no relationship at all between the vaginal abnormalities in female children and the mothers' use of DES during pregnancy. The action of excluding fertile women from exposure to DES or preventing pregnant women from using it therapeutically was based on the best evidence available at that time, and it was obviously the most prudent approach to take. Should we have waited nine years for contradictory evidence to be developed without invoking restrictive or exclusionary actions? Suppose that evidence never came into being? We could have exposed many people unnecessarily to an agent with possible life-threatening effects. What would your decision have been nine years ago? That is the type of decision that employers are and will be faced with every day in the future. What will your decision be?

## Discussion

**Richard H. Egdahl:** Jeanne Stellman, how do you feel on this issue? Would you change the policy Dr. Clyne describes with respect to restricting pregnant women from areas where certain exposure limits are exceeded?

**Jeanne M. Stellman:** I'd really need to see a list of the chemicals and exposure levels we're talking about, because there is not universal agreement on safe limits. I do not advocate putting women into workplaces where they are exposed to things that will damage the fetus, and I think there are other social solutions available. I don't know how the Cyanamid plant in question is organized. There may be ten departments where there are safe jobs and one department with unsafe jobs, so that there may be other options for the women who work there. If the choice is between working in that particular plant and department versus unemployment, that would be something else again. I would have to be fairly certain that we weren't just pulling fertile women out and leaving other workers exposed. If we agree with Dr. Clyne that a given level of exposure is safe for everybody else and that there is a real risk for the fetus, then it may be a reasonable policy. I am not arguing for carte blanche rules that say women should never be excluded from anything.

**Robert M. Clyne:** American Cyanamid gave women at our Willow Island plant* the alternative of moving to other jobs at no loss of pay, to

---

*In September 1978 American Cyanamid Company instituted a policy at its Willow Island Plant in West Virginia which excluded women with childbearing potential (under age 50) from working in areas of the plant where they would be exposed to lead. According to the *Wall Street Journal* (January 3, 1979, p. 16), lawsuits have been filed by five women who allege that they were pressured to undergo sterilization procedures in order to avoid transfer to lower paying jobs. Cyanamid disagrees, saying that they offered bid in on other production jobs within a three-month period of time, and they preferred the job that we transferred them to. Two of the women were allowed to move back into the original area because they of their own choice have been sterilized. Then they started all of this fuss and furor. It's astounding just how complex this problem is—from the legal standpoint, from a moral standpoint, from the standpoint of doing what we have been trained to do and that is to protect the employee in his or her workplace. Our company, which is not as big as DuPont, has 2,000 products which require some 20,000 different chemicals to manufacture. We don't have all the information that we need, and I am terrified to hear that we may get into the ballgame of not allowing anybody any exposure until we have done a sufficient amount of toxicological work to assure that there is *no* risk in the workplace. This to me would mean that we halt everything in the United States for x number of years to develop that information, assuming that we had the toxicological facilities in which to do it. If we require expensive modifications that cannot be passed on to the consumer, what will eventually happen is that moderately profitable processes will cease to be profitable. Then neither women nor men will be eligible for the jobs there, because there won't be any jobs.

relocation at comparable pay to all female workers displaced by the exclusion and discouraged sterilization as a solution. Other large corporations (e.g., General Motors, Olin Corporation, Allied Chemical) have also established similiar protection through exclusion measures.

# The Control of Hazardous Exposures in the Workplace

*Edward J. Bernacki, M.D.*

# 13

The goal of occupational medicine is to prevent injury and illness in the workplace. This is achieved by separating the susceptible person from a disease-producing substance, usually by reducing the concentration of such substances to safe levels through engineering (environmental) controls. If this approach is not adequate, personal protective equipment is usually the next step. Actual removal of the worker from the offending environment is resorted to only after all other methods have failed to guarantee safety.

To select the proper type of control (engineering, personal protection, or worker removal), two steps are necessary: identifying and quantifying the risks of the workplace, and assessing the capacity of individuals to work safety in the environment. If lack of information makes these steps impossible—if not enough is known about the hazards of a work environment or about the health status of the person who wishes to work in that environment—and if existing or planned environmental controls are inadequate to assure safety, then removal of the worker is the only recourse available to guarantee safety. While the option of removing or not permitting a worker to enter certain environments is considered an industrial hygiene failure, it still must be used in situations where our information is inadequate. Unfortunately, this situation is rather common because, first, industrial toxicology is a new and relatively unstudied field, and second, there are too few occupational health professionals performing the environmental or personal evaluations necessary to quantify the hazards.

Interest in studying occupational disease has only recently been rekindled. Most of the information now used to determine the potential health effects of many occupational hazards dates from the 1920s and 1930s. This means that limited, outdated information is employed to predict the deleterious effects of many occupational agents on adult workers and on developing embryos and fetuses inadvertantly placed in the work environment. How most chemical agents affect a worker's body and reproductive cells and how they affect fetuses is simply not known. Coupled with this lack is a lack of information on the dose of an agent necessary to produce disease or cause injury. In only a few instances does valid information exist on dose effect–response relationships of industrial agents and in even fewer instances are good exposure effect–response relationships available. With few exceptions, dose and exposure effect–response relationships are derived from animal data, poisoning episodes, or case studies on one or a handful of workers. These are certainly inadequate to set and define sensible threshold limit values.

The second problem we face in instituting engineering or personal protection controls is the number of assessments in a given environment needed to identify hazards, evaluate worker susceptibility, and characterize exposures. This situation is due primarily to an inadequate supply of industrial hygienists to perform environmental evaluations and of occupational physicians to interpret the significance of the findings. Even in corporations that employ a great many of these professionals, only a few work environments can be studied in any great detail.

The last deficiency which forces the use of worker removal as a control strategy is the nonuniversality of performing preplacement and follow-up physical examinations on persons who have been or will be exposed to hazardous agents. This is due, again, to an undersupply of professionals trained to do these evaluations, as well as to the unwillingness of many employers to add a physical examination to the hiring process.

Evaluating an individual and the working environment and selecting the best control method to assure safety, even if it be worker removal, is a preventive medical strategy which is, I feel, consistent with equal opportunity legislation. Title VII of the Civil Rights Act prohibits discrimination in employment on the basis of sex alone,[1] but if the preferences and abilities of individual women are taken into account when making placement decisions, sex discrimination can be avoided.[2] Individual susceptibilities can only be assessed by a thorough physical examination, preferably done by a physician familiar with work-related hazards.

When performing such an examination, the physician may elicit information about previous reproductive failures, the desire to have children, hysterectomies, and other relevant issues. Using this information, along with knowledge of the workplace, the physician can assess current and potential risk to a female or her fetus and choose the appropriate control measure. The use of multiple parameters in making the decision avoids any need to refuse a woman a particular job simply because she is female or because she may eventually become pregnant. This procedure treats males and females equally, enabling employers to hire the most qualified person for a particular job. This guarantees the safety of the employee and the fetus to the maximum extent possible.

In its attempts to assure a safe and healthful working environment, OSHA requires, with few exceptions, the elimination of exposure potential through engineering controls.[3] In the OSHA construct the work environment must be altered so that the most susceptible person or organism can be placed in it without harm. This, of course, is a goal worth pursuing, and it is logical and defensible for agents whose toxicities and whose exposure effect-response relationships are known. However, these facts are not known for most actual or potential workplace hazards. And thus the dilemma cannot be resolved until more information about workplace hazards can be obtained.

## NOTES

1. M. N. Hilton, "The National Scene," *Journal of Occupational Medicine* 16 (1974): 535–538.
2. Ibid.; and J. S. Ward, "Sex Discrimination Is Essential in Industry," *Journal of Occupational Medicine* 20 (1978): 594–596.
3. A. Sloan, "Employer's Tort Liability When a Female Is Exposed to Harmful Substances," *Employees Relations Law Journal* (1978): 506–515.

# PREGNANCY AND MATERNITY LEAVE

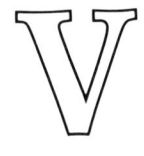

V

# A Legal Perspective on Pregnancy Leave and Benefits

*Nina G. Stillman, J.D.*

# 14

Over the last fourteen years, pregnancy benefits issues have proved to be a surprisingly fertile ground for litigation. Specifically, there has been a host of administrative agency and court actions involving, in one form or another, the question of whether employers may accord differential benefit treatment to pregnancy—as compared with other "traditional" temporary disabilities—without violating the sex discrimination prohibition contained in Title VII of the Civil Rights Act of 1964, as amended ("Title VII").[1]

The almost obsessive interest displayed by discrimination agencies, the courts, employers, and workers with respect to this issue is particularly curious in light of the anomolous fashion in which the sex discrimination prohibition was included in the bill that eventually became Title VII. There was no language in Title VII itself when enacted that in any way referred to pregnancy; nor was there anything in the legislative history underlying the sex discrimination prohibition that equated discrimination on the basis of pregnancy with discrimination on the basis of sex. Indeed, almost no legislative history was generated with respect to the sex discrimination prohibition. This is partly the result of the provision's having been added at the last minute by a group of southern Congressmen in an attempt to defeat passage of the bill.[2] In fact, several of the leading proponents of the bill spoke in opposition to the sex discrimination amendment.[3] More significantly, every male member of the House who voiced support for inclusion of the sex discrimination prohibition into the bill ultimately voted against its passage.[4]

It is also worthy of note that the Equal Employment Opportunity Commission, the federal agency that administers and enforces Title VII, came rather late to the cause of pregnancy discrimination as sex discrimination. When the EEOC first issued its Guidelines on Discrimination Because of Sex on November 24, 1965,[5] no view was expressed with regard to the treatment of pregnancy-related disabilities. Nor was such a view set out in either the Guidelines' February 21, 1968, amendments[6] or August 19, 1969, amendments.[7] In fact, it was not until the April 5, 1972,[8] version of the Guidelines that the matter was expressly addressed. In the 1972 Guidelines, the EEOC espoused the position that Title VII mandates that pregnancy disabilities be accorded the same benefit treatment as any other temporary disability. In so holding, the EEOC made a complete about-face from an earlier interpretation of the law contained in a 1966 opinion letter of the EEOC General Counsel.[9]

In view of the EEOC's waffling, as well as the major financial commitment that full pregnancy benefit coverage would entail for employers, it was inevitable that the issue of whether pregnancy disabilities must be accorded the same benefit treatment as other disabilities under Title VII would eventually reach the United States Supreme Court. The case that everyone concerned hoped would resolve the question once and for all was *General Electric Company v. Gilbert.*[10] To the surprise of many, the Supreme Court in this decision rejected the EEOC's 1972 position, which had been adopted by many lower courts, that it was unlawful sex discrimination to exclude pregnancy-related disabilities from employer-provided disability insurance, i.e., wage continuation, plans. Unfortunately, the *General Electric* decision raised more questions than it answered. Employers elected to follow a broad interpretation of the decision, seeing in it support for the proposition that distinctions based on pregnancy are not unlawful sex discrimination in themselves unless they could be shown to be a pretext or a subterfuge for intentional sex discrimination. The EEOC and employees, not surprisingly, adopted a very narrow reading of *General Electric* which was set forth in an EEOC directive to its field offices.[11] Nor were the unresolved issues laid to rest in the Supreme Court's next pregnancy decision, *Nashville Gas Company v. Satty*,[12] which was issued exactly one year to the day after *General Electric*.

As a result of the extremely negative reaction to the Supreme Court's *General Electric* decision on the part of the unions, feminists, and many liberal Congressmen, several bills were introduced to amend Title VII expressly to cover pregnancy. To this end, on October 31, 1978, the Pregnancy Disability Law[13] was enacted.

## The Pregnancy Disability Law of 1978

The new pregnancy law amends the Civil Rights Act of 1964 by making the Title VII prohibition of sex discrimination in employment specifically applicable to discrimination against pregnant women.* The law provides in part that:

> ... women affected by pregnancy, childbirth, or related medical conditions shall be treated the same for all employment-related purposes, including receipt of benefits under fringe benefit programs, as other persons not so affected but similar in their ability or inability to work ....

Fundamentally, therefore, the new law prohibits employers from treating the health problems or disabilities arising from pregnancy differently from similar health problems or disabilities caused by illness or injury. With regard to fringe benefits such as disability leave or insurance, the law does not require employers to provide such benefits to pregnant women if they are not provided for other disabilities; rather, the law requires employers to provide benefits to pregnant women on the same terms and conditions that they offer them, if at all, to other employees.

The new law further provides that employers may not reduce existing benefits during the first year after enactment in order to comply

---

*The Pregnancy Disability Law amends the Civil Rights Act of 1964 by adding a new subsection (k) to Section 701 which provides as follows:

> (k) The terms "because of sex" or "on the basis of sex" include, but are not limited to, because of or on the basis of pregnancy, childbirth or related medical conditions; and women affected by pregnancy, childbirth, or related medical conditions shall be treated the same for all employment-related purposes, including receipt of benefits under fringe benefit programs, as other persons not so affected but similar in their ability or inability to work, and nothing in section 703(h) of this title shall be interpreted to permit otherwise. This subsection shall not require an employer to pay for health insurance benefits for abortion, except where the life of the mother would be endangered if the fetus were carried to term, or except where medical complications have arisen from an abortion: Provided, that nothing herein shall preclude an employer from providing abortion benefits or otherwise affect bargaining agreements in regard to abortion.

with the law's requirements, even though the cost of providing such benefits may be substantially increased by the addition of pregnancy coverage.* However, where benefits are subject to a collective bargaining agreement, the moratorium on reduction extends to the expiration of the collective bargaining agreement even if that occurs after October 31, 1979.**

Under the new law, employers need only cover pregnant employees under existing disability benefit programs for the period of actual disability. Thus, if a pregnant employee wishes to take an early pregnancy leave prior to the onset of any debilitating symptoms or if she elects to remain home after her recovery in order to take care of her child, she is not entitled to use sick leave, either paid or unpaid, and the employer is not obligated to pay out disability, i.e., wage continuation, benefits. Under such circumstances, the employee would be required to utilize her personal leave or vacation for the time off when she was not actually disabled.

Finally, the new law provides that employers are not obligated "to pay for health insurance benefits for abortions, except where the life of the mother would be endangered if the fetus were carried to term or except where medical complications have arisen from an abortion. . . ." Employers are, of course, in no way precluded from offering full coverage for abortions. Moreover, while employers are not required to pay health insurance for nontherapeutic abortions, they may not deny sick leave or other disability benefits for the time spent away from work because of an abortion. Similarly, employers may not refuse to hire a woman merely because she has had an abortion. Nor may she be fired or otherwise disciplined for "contemplating" or exercising her constitutionally guaranteed right to have an abortion.[14]

## Whither Goest Pregnancy Law?

The Pregnancy Disability Law has already had and will continue to have a profound impact on the employment relationship. While its effects can be seen at all levels of the employment cycle, from hiring to retirement, perhaps its most significant impact has been in the area of pregnancy benefits and leave.

Prior to enactment of the law, many employers did not allow pregnant employees to utilize paid or unpaid sick leave, short-term disa-

---

*If the benefit plans are contributory between employers and employees, employees generally—not merely women or pregnant employees—will have to pay their usual share of the increased cost.

**However, even after the moratorium on benefit reduction expires, if an employer is found to have violated Title VII, as now amended, by providing greater benefits to one sex, such employer will not be permitted to lower existing benefits as a means of correcting the discrimination.

bility insurance, or accrued paid and unpaid sick days for time off owing to pregnancy.* Instead, the general practice was to offer a fairly liberal *unpaid* pregnancy leave which could extend anywhere from four months to a year. Customarily, such pregnancy leaves did not require proof of disability or other documentation. Indeed, these leaves were not even contingent upon disability, but instead could be applied to both the prebirth and postbirth periods. In some cases, employers would allow a flat six weeks' disability insurance coverage for time off owing to pregnancy even though all other nonoccupational disabilities were covered for a period of, for example, up to thirteen, twenty-six, or fifty-two weeks.

It is now clear that implementation of the new law has engendered a profound change in the traditional concept of the pregnancy leave. First, pregnant employees will no longer have the liberal time off, albeit generally unpaid time off, that was formerly available to them. Instead, pregnant employees are now limited by the requirements of the applicable sick leave policy as well as their own actual disability. Although pregnant employees may now receive disability benefits coverage for pregnancy, they must be "actually disabled" in order to collect benefits. It is crucial to remember that the mere fact of being pregnant will not entitle an employee to disability coverage; rather, she must be disabled by her pregnancy before coverage is appropriate. As the House Committee Report states:

> The only time the employer will be required to allow pregnant workers to use this leave [i.e., paid sick leave] is during the time they are medically unable to work, during the same period of time and under the same terms applicable to other employee [sic]. For example, if a woman wants to stay home to take care of the child, no benefit must be paid because this is not a medically determined condition related to pregnancy. And, if an employer has a temporary disability program which pays up to 15 weeks (as 90 percent of disability plans provide for 15 to 26 weeks) that does not mean a pregnant worker can receive benefits for all of those 15 weeks. She may only receive benefits for those weeks during which she is medically unable to work. Testimony before the Committee indicates that in 95 percent of the cases, the time lost from work due to pregnancy is 6 weeks or less, so barring any medical complications, this period would be the normal time a pregnant woman would be covered. If, however, medical complications arose, which is the case in about 5 percent of all pregnancies, these complications

---

*Sick leave is time off from work owing to illness or injury; it can be either paid or unpaid time. Short-term disability insurance (also known as sickness and accident insurance) is a wage continuation plan for employees off from work owing to nonoccupational illness or injury. Accrued sick days are a certain number of days allowed each year for time off owing to illness or injury. Some employers offer both paid and unpaid sick days. Some employers allow the accrual of sick days from one year to the other. Sick day plans are usually found in banks, law firms, schools, retail establishments, and other white collar employment settings.

should be covered by the same time limits or dollar amounts otherwise provided disabled workers.[15]

A second change in the traditional concept of the pregnancy leave is that employees who are not disabled but who wish to take time off prior to the onset of labor or for child care purposes after the birth may now only take such time off pursuant to an available personal leave or vacation plan. It must be remembered, however, that employers who are willing to offer a child care leave for new mothers must also make such a leave available to new fathers. And, in fact, several employers, including American Telephone & Telegraph Co., have already announced that they will offer child care leaves for both new mothers and new fathers.[16]

A third change which is now being observed in the concept of pregnancy leave involves reporting requirements. In the past, employers usually required pregnant employees to report their condition and obtain certification from the personal physician with respect to the expected date of birth, the expected date for leave commencement, and whether the particular employee was physically fit and able to continue working. Once the employee went on leave she may also have been required to report when she intended to return to active employment and to provide a note from her personal physician releasing her for work.

With the new law mandating that employers provide disability benefits for time off owing to pregnancy disability, employers are now implementing stricter reporting requirements designed to determine, to the extent possible, whether the pregnant employee is actually disabled and thereby entitled to benefits coverage. However, before employers proceed in such a fashion, they should keep several factors in mind. First, any reporting requirements must be applied in a nondiscriminatory manner, i.e., pregnancy cannot be singled out for more burdensome reporting obligations than other disabilities. Thus, should an employer wish to continue its prior policy of requiring pregnant employees to report their conditions, they should consider formulating a policy to cover all anticipated disabilities. An example of such a nondiscriminatory policy might be as follows:

### Policy

In order for the company better to protect the health of its employees and administer any benefits for which they may be eligible, employees who develop physical conditions which may foreseeably lessen their ability safely to perform their job duties must immediately report the existence of such a condition to _____. Examples of such conditions are diabetes, epilepsy, angina pectoris, and pregnancy.

Employees reporting such conditions must obtain certification from their personal physician which should include:
1. the nature of the condition;
2. whether, in the physician's opinion, the condition will require the curtailment, modification, or discontinuation of current job duties and, if so, why;
3. whether surgery or hospitalization is imminent;
4. whether the employee is on a maintenance drug such as insulin;
5. in the case of pregnancy, the expected date of childbirth and, when the date for discontinuation of work owing to pregnancy differs from the expected date of childbirth, the date on which the pregnant employee should discontinue working and the reason why such data differs from the expected date of childbirth.*

Another consideration for employers to keep in mind when developing a disability reporting policy is how frequently the employee will be required to provide certification as to continued disability. It is probably both onerous and unrealistic to expect an employee on pregnancy leave to provide weekly reports from her personal physician attesting to continued disability. As a matter of convenience, employers may instead wish to have a set period of time, such as five or six weeks, which may elapse before the reporting requirements become operative. However, it must be remembered that the requirements should be applied to all disabilities. A six-week reporting moratorium may, thus, be too liberal in the case of other non–pregnancy-related disabilities. Under such circumstances, the employer should explore structuring its policy in such a fashion that the frequency of reporting will be at the discretion of the employer, based on the nature and severity of the disability.

A stricter reporting policy for employees on pregnancy leave is probably the primary method employers have at their disposal to control what they fear will be an abuse of the pregnancy disability benefit. Many employers believe—rightly or wrongly—that pregnant employees will claim they are disabled in order to receive lengthy paid disability leaves. These employers also believe that most personal physicians will happily provide their patients with the necessary certification on the theory that it is always better if their pregnant patients can stay off the job and rest without the loss of substantial wages. While

---

*As an alternative to the second paragraph of the sample policy, employers may wish merely to use the following:

Employees reporting such conditions must pick up at _____ a questionnaire to be filled out by the personal physician and returned within ____ days to _____ .

employers generally are not too optimistic, it is hoped that the more specific character of the inquiries to the personal physician and the frequent reporting required of the employee, as well as the knowledge that the reports will be reviewed by the company medical director, will have a moderating influence both on the personal physician and the pregnant employee. Certainly this will not happen overnight. Indeed, there will probably be a rather lengthy and painful period of adjustment to the new law for all parties concerned.

A fourth change in the traditional concept of the pregnancy leave with which employers must now contend is how to avoid turning the paid leave into an additional form of severance. In 1973, during the trial of the *General Electric* case, evidence was introduced by the employer that 40 percent of all employees who took maternity leave did not return to work, whereas 99 percent of all employees on sick leave did return.

Whether such statistics are accurate for today is open to question. Clearly, there have been noticeable changes throughout the 1970s which indicate that more women are continuing to work after childbirth. Inflation is perhaps the primary influence for keeping mothers in the work force. The consciousness-raising of the feminist movement is another. Nevertheless, there are still significant numbers of young women who have no intention of returning to work after their children are born. In the past, such women usually informed their employer of their intention, but the new law provides a disincentive for such honesty.

It is now highly unlikely that a pregnant employee will tell her employer of an intention not to return, since it will mean forfeiting benefits for the period of her pregnancy-related disability. Such understandable reticence creates several problems. First, under the law, the employer must keep open the job of an employee on leave owing to pregnancy. If the employee does not tell the employer that she does not intend to return to work, the employer cannot make arrangements to fill the vacant position. This creates substantial labor planning problems. Second, the employee who does not intend to return is, in reality, drawing extra, unjustified severance pay. The purpose of disability benefits is to assist an injured or sick employee financially so that he or she can recover without undue anxiety and return to work as soon as possible. It is a benefit designed to maintain employee continuity. Any employee who has no intention of returning to work should not be entitled to disability benefits.

Unfortunately, there does not now appear to be a satisfactory solution to this dilemma. One approach would be to pay the disability benefits only after the employee has returned to work for a set period of time. However, such a policy could result in severe hardship for a truly disabled employee who needs the wage supplement during the period of illness or injury. Moreover, it would defeat the whole purpose of the disability benefit.

A fifth change brought on by the new pregnancy law which surfaced almost immediately after April 29, 1979, involves the interaction of the new law's requirements with the problem of occupational fetotoxicity. This problem is exemplified by the experience of the radiology profession. Traditionally, pregnant x-ray technicians were placed on unpaid maternity leave as soon as their condition was detected in order to avoid injury to the fetus through radiation exposure. The question that now predominates is whether the pregnant x-ray technician is entitled to disability benefits for the duration of her pregnancy, childbirth, and recovery? It is arguable that the pregnant employee is not truly disabled—in the sense that her physical condition has not rendered her *unable* to perform her job duties—and, therefore, is not entitled to disability benefits. However, it may also be argued that she is disabled—in the sense that her physical condition makes her unable to perform her job *safely*—and, therefore, is entitled to disability benefits.

The importance of the problem is obvious: On the one hand you have the employer who is usually a doctor or a group of doctors. As doctors they are acutely aware of the danger to the health of the fetus; as employers they are deeply concerned about paying disability benefits for what could be a nine-month period while at the same time keeping the job open for the duration of the leave. On the other hand, you have the healthy pregnant employee who faces nine months of unpaid leave.

In some cases, the pregnant employee desires to continue working and offers to provide the employer a waiver of liability. Unfortunately, such a waiver cannot bind the ultimately born child or its father from later suing the employer for any injuries which may arguably have resulted from the mother's occupational radiation exposure. In other cases, the employer has determined that the occupational exposures are so far below the 0.5-rems dose limit recommended for the fetus by the National Council on Radiation Protection and Measurements[17] that the risk to the fetus is minimal. However, employers opting for this approach must remember the risk from possible leaks or other equipment failure which could lead to sudden massive exposures.

The foregoing should not in any way be viewed as a comprehensive analysis of the 1978 Pregnancy Disability Law and its impact. Rather, it is merely a very brief discussion of the genesis of the new law and how its provisions affect one aspect of the pregnancy issue, that is, the pregnancy leave. Indeed, there are many other areas which can and should be explored, such as the law's impact on pregnant dependents and on retirees, the extent of the prohibition on benefits reduction, the interjection by the EEOC in Question and Answer 12 of the handicap discrimination laws' "reasonable accommodation" principle, etc. These, as well as yet-to-surface questions, should continue to keep the pregnancy issue a significant source of concern and litigation for employers, employees, organized labor, the government, and the medical community.

## NOTES

1. 42 U.S.C. §2000e et seq. Title VII prohibits covered employers from discriminating against individuals on the basis of race, color, religion, sex, or national origin.
2. 110 Cong. Rec. 2577 (1964); see also Comment, Civil Rights Act of 1964: An Exception To Prohibitions on Employment Discrimination, 55 Iowa L. Rev. 509, 511 (1969); Note: Discrimination in Employment: An Attempt to Interpret Title VII of the Civil Rights Act of 1964, 1968 Duke L. J. 671, 676 n. 35 (hereafter cited as "1968 Duke L. J.").
3. 110 Cong. Rec. 2577–2584 (1964). Among those speaking in opposition to the amendment were Representatives Celler (D.–N.Y.), chairman of the House Committee on the Judiciary, Roosevelt (D.–Cal.), Green (D.–Ore.), and Lindsey (R.–N.Y.).
4. 110 Cong. Rec. 15897 (1964). See also 55 Iowa L. Rev. at 512; 1968 Duke L. J. at 677.
5. 30 Fed. Reg. 14926.
6. 33 Fed. Reg. 3344.
7. 34 Fed. Reg. 13367.
8. 37 Fed. Reg. 6835.
9. This EEOC opinion letter, dated November 15, 1966, was identified and placed into evidence by former EEOC General Counsel Charles Duncan during the trial of *Gilbert v. General Electric Company*, 375 F. Supp. 367 (E. D. Va. 1974), aff'd., 519 F.2d 661 (4th Cir. 1975), rev'd., 429 U.S. 125 (1976). It stated, in part, that:

    > The Commission's policy with respect to pregnancy does not seek to compare an employer's treatment of illness or injury with his treatment of maternity, since maternity is a temporary disability unique to the female sex and more or less to be anticipated during the working life of most women employees . . . We do not believe that an employer must provide the same fringe benefits for pregnancy as he provides for illness.

10. 429 U.S. 125 (1976).
11. See EEOC directive to its field offices, 1977 DLR no. 10, pp. A-9 to A-11 (Jan. 14, 1977), which states that EEOC would find that an employer violates Title VII by:
    - refusing to hire, train, assign or promote pregnant women;
    - refusing to hire, train, assign or promote married women;

- refusing to hire, assign or promote women of childbearing age;
- enforcing mandatory maternity leaves for predetermined periods;
- discharging pregnant women;
- denying reemployment rights to women on leave for pregnancy-related reasons;
- denying unemployment benefits to pregnant women;
- denying seniority of longevity credit to women on leave for pregnancy-related reasons;
- denying accrued leave to pregnant women who have worked less than a stated time period;
- paying of lower periodic amounts to retired women according to sex-segregated actuarial tables;
- denying disability or medical benefits for disabilities which are unrelated to pregnancy or childbirth, whether or not they occur during a pregnancy, childbirth, or recovery from childbirth.

12. 434 U.S. 136 (1977). In the *Satty* decision, the Court addressed itself to two issues. First, it held that an employer did not violate Title VII by denying employees the right to utilize accrued paid sick leave for pregnancy. Second, it held that Title VII was violated when an employer denied accumulated seniority to employees returning from a pregnancy leave.
13. P. L. 95–555, 92 Stat. 2076 (1978).
14. See Questions and Answers 34–37 of the "Guidelines on Sex Discrimination: Adoption of Final Interpretative Guidelines and Questions and Answers," 44 Fed. Reg. 23804 (April 20, 1979).
15. H. R. Report no. 95–948, 95th Cong., 2d Sess. (1978): 5.
16. See "AT&T Replacing Maternity Program for Its Employees," *Wall Street Journal* (April 23, 1979): 32.
17. See *Guidelines On Pregnancy And Work*, American College of Obstetricians and Gynecologists and National Institute for Occupational Safety and Health (Sept. 1977): 23; and *Review of NCRP Radiation Dose Limit for Embryo and Fetus in Occupationally Exposed Women*, National Council on Radiation Protection and Measurements, Report no. 53, Washington, D.C., 1977.

# Discussion

**Eleanor Tilson:** The pregnancy law is a major victory because the coverage of maternity disability has hitherto been very ineffective for most working women. If they became ill or suffered complications, their chances of collecting for disability were virtually nil. The law is clearly an advance in that it makes it possible for women to collect maternity disability. The issue of leave is separate.

**Iver S. Ravin:** We tend to lose sight of one dimension of this. Pregnancy benefits are a social benefit as much as if not more than a medical benefit. If it's a great victory for women that they got the bill passed, it's an equally great victory for their husbands or for whoever supports them, because pregnancy is a family event. At least it was when my wife was pregnant. I was a doctor just starting in practice, and when my wife left her job with no benefits, our income dropped precipitously. We are talking, really, about the transfer of funds, because the rates that AT&T's or Boston Edison's customers pay are what ultimately pays for the pregnancy benefits. Nobody is getting anything for nothing.

**Tilson:** I certainly agree that the maternity law is a victory for the family and not just for women. I accept that amendment.

**Robert N. Clyne:** I have another concern. If, as has been suggested, the chief concern of the practicing physician is to keep his private patients happy with him, I can see his role in certifying disability being abused brutally. The corporate physician is caught on the horns of a dilemma. Suppose the private physician says a patient ought to be off for five or six months but the corporate physician overrules that. If she aborts or something, then he's in real trouble. But the woman may have gone to Dr. Jones seven or eight months into her pregnancy and said, "I don't feel like working on the assembly line. My belly protrudes, and I've got to lean over and twist the bolt or whatever." What is the doctor going to do? Whether or not she's disabled, he'll write the note. So we're hooked. Now if that's an advance for society, I'd like to go back to the Dark Ages.

**Donna J. Morrison:** I'm sure all occupational doctors are knowledgeable in what will and will not harm the fetus. But I think it's reasonable to assume that the average obstetrician has no knowledge of the work environment at all and will therefore err on the side of caution by encouraging female patients to stay away from occupational exposures, especially with the news media publicizing all the types of exposure there may be. There is going to be a problem, but we should acknowledge that it might not be just because obstetricians don't dare dissuade a woman patient from taking time off to relax in a country club atmosphere. It might be rather that they're greatly concerned about her health and the health of the fetus and are going to be cautious. The question that I have, since I really don't deal in this area, is what is the biggest problem? Is it that management sincerely feels that women are going to abuse this system? If so, what is the statistical basis for feeling that women are going to abuse this any more than the average person will abuse any type of insurance program?

**Tilson:** I take exception to the assumption that women are going to abuse this benefit. I think most firms will use good sense and good judgment in applying the law and women won't abuse it. New York State has had a maternity law for almost two years, and there has not been the abuse that many predicted when that law first came on the books.

**Bruce W. Karrh:** My view is conditioned by the fact that I've practiced medicine on both sides of the street, having been in private practice for a while in a small town where I did obstetrics along with everything else. At that time my obligation was to the patient: it was the patient who may or may not pay me, who may or may not sue me for malpractice, and if she wanted to take a week off from work, fine—it didn't bother me and it may have helped her. I had no obligation whatsoever to the employer. Also, I found that patients would exaggerate the job demands, telling me that the job required certain things that in fact it didn't. And it's not really a malicious thing; it's just they would pick out the worst part of the job and say that's what their job was. And then when I went with industry I found myself in the opposite role, trying to get people back to work when they were no longer disabled. There are no incentives on the practicing physician to do other than take the easy way out. I did when I was in practice. So we're really going to have a problem with pregnancy leave and it's going to require very careful control and careful consideration.

**Jeanne M. Stellman:** There are always abuses in this world and people who don't abuse. That's the price we pay for having a society that says that working people have some rights and benefits. In professions where women have been able to get enjoyable, rewarding jobs that pay well, they fight to stay on the job as long as they possibly can and come back as soon as they can. Women who have alienating jobs may want to try to get out of work.

**Glen Wegner:** How long the disability lasts is not only a question of the physical aspects, "I don't feel well," or "I'm tired," or "I feel I've got varicose veins," or whatever. There is also the important psychological aspect of a mother's need to be with a child and vice versa for the period immediately postpartum.

**Stellman:** Pregnancy as a legal issue has been around for a good ten years, and will have to be around for another five or ten years if we're really going to go to the root of the social problems. A lot now depends upon the present administration and the state of the economy over the next ten years, to be very pragmatic. Several other issues right now have precedence in Congress. Congress feels they've done their bit in passing this law, and I doubt they'll soon be ready to rethink it.

This has been a hard-fought struggle, with many compromises: the abortion compromise was just one; the concept of pregnancy as a disability was, in a sense, another. Three top women at the congressional hearings who testified said pregnancy is not an illness but there is a period during pregnancy when you have disabling conditions. Obviously, when you are in labor, you're disabled. People aren't saying that normal pregnancy is a disability in old-fashioned terms such that the woman goes and hides herself like a leper, but because certain aspects of pregnancy are disabling we must treat it as a disability. It's a matter of convenience to use that terminology. We have no other terminology, and people are familiar with the term *disability*. The problem with the term is how do you differentiate pregnancy from true disability? I'm not sure I see an answer. But I think it's important to reiterate what Nina Stillman has said: this is an antidiscrimination law, it's social policy only in the negative sense. It's not a positive construction of social policy with respect to pregnancy.

**Edward J. Bernacki:** Many women have difficulty performing their jobs because of pregnancy, but the question arises who should determine whether the pregnant female can or cannot perform her job? It is my belief that the individual best able to evaluate the health risk of a pregnancy or its complications is the female worker's obstetrician. Advice regarding the effects of environmental agents both chemical and physical on the pregnant female or her fetus is best received from an occupational physician familiar with the worker's job. Consequently, the source of the disability is the best indicator of who should decide the appropriateness of work restrictions. If the reason for work modification arises out of the pregnancy itself, without regard to the environment, the responsible person is the employee's personal physician. Limitations based on workplace considerations and not on complications of pregnancy are the responsibility of the occupational physician and he or she alone should make that decision.

**John L. Bauer:** One of the first cases that occurred at Armco under the new law caused us some concern. Before April 29 we granted a maternity leave of absence and a six-week disability benefit paid in a lump sum. When the first pregnant employee under the new plan came to us we explained that she could begin a leave but she would not be paid disability benefits until she was certified disabled from performing the duties of her job by a licensed physician. These benefits would continue for as long as her doctor certified her as being disabled. She seemed to understand, yet a month later she returned saying she had just seen her doctor. She didn't realize she was supposed to be disabled when she initially came in. This gave us great concern since in effect she was saying she couldn't tell she was disabled. This of course is quite different from how we typically define a disability.

We've become very sensitive to potential abuse problems in this area. We've now established guidelines that if the disability exceeds eight weeks with no apparent complications, we encourage our plant physician to call the attending physician to work out problems with a minimum of paper work. We fully expect it's going to be a year or so before this is worked out. It's going to be a long-term educational process for our female employees as well as the physicians.

**Stellman:** Of course, Armco Steel is not where the typical woman works; that's the issue.

**Tilson:** In the department store industry, we are dealing with the issue of maternity disability as we would with any other disability. With a doctor's statement that there are no complications, eight weeks is a normal maternity disability. It can be postpartum, antepartum, or both. If a doctor's form comes in indicating that the woman is unable to work for four months, we will send that woman for an evaluation to establish whether she indeed cannot work. We apply the same yardstick for maternity disability that we do for any other disability. Should a man working in a department store be disabled for a hernia, we have a yardstick for how long that disability should last, and so we feel we are within our province to make a parallel determination for maternity leave. And we do not see any excesses. Women in fact are working longer. The normal disability of eight weeks is more than ample to cover their needs in most cases, so we do not see many problems. The issue of the leave of absence has been negotiated through the collective bargaining process, and six months' leave of absence was established.

**Nina G. Stillman:** Here's the crunch. Most industries are willing to be fairly liberal with regard to pregnancies and to use a rule of thumb without questioning the woman. But they're going to have to question her unless they want to take the same approach with all disabilities—the guy with the hernia or with the history of angina. Do you want him reporting only once within a ten-week period? Typically, he has to report once every two weeks. You've got a reverse discrimination problem. That's why Ellie Tilson's plan of eight weeks for pregnancy to use any way you want isn't going to work unless the Storeworkers' Union Trust is willing to say anyone with any disability can have the same eight weeks.

**Tilson:** The concept is that someone is entitled to eight weeks as a normal disability, and we will not question or send for an evaluation.

**Stillman:** And that's across the board for males or females?

**Tilson:** It depends upon the illness—for a hernia or a heart condition it would be longer, obviously. But across the board, we do the same thing in any disability. Claims for men who do the heavy shipping and packing and incur back injuries, again, will get a doctor's evaluation once the time has exceeded a preestablished guideline for back injuries.

**William E. R. Greer:** Gillette's policy is very liberal. One of the significant factors is the continued salary policy for the Gillette employee throughout the disability, as long as he or she is going to come back to work sometime. The policy will now probably be rewritten, but it has been that once a worker knew she was pregnant and reported that to us, we sent a letter to her obstetrician describing the nature of her work and requesting the expected date of delivery plus work restrictions. We hoped that we would stimulate the obstetrician to look at the job demands in his or her evaluation, although we know full well that most obstetricians probably don't. In any event, she was allowed two weeks before delivery and six weeks after, as an informal sort of understanding. Of course, she had disability possibilities beyond that.

We have our problems, such as an obstetrician who requested pregnancy disability for a woman who worked on the thirty-seventh floor, saying she couldn't travel in elevators during her pregnancy. Our lawyers insisted that we go along with that, although I couldn't see how this woman was truly disabled. But if she'd come back to work at our instigation and then miscarried, we would have been responsible. Women are often tired early in their pregnancies. But is that a disability? Many doctors are going to say they think she's very tired, too tired to work, and therefore disabled. How do you reconcile that with other workers who may also be tired, working two jobs or something? Can you say to the pregnant woman, "All right, you're very tired for the first three hours in the morning, so you work in the second shift." We once tried that, but the woman decided she'd rather not work. I've sent letters to local obstetricians in three problem cases and they have answered none of them. I didn't really expect them to, but I sent them anyway. It's difficult to handle some of these pregnancy cases; in medicine or surgery I have no difficulty in dealing with the attending physician, but I'm a lot less sure about disability in these ambiguous pregnancy situations. This policy's been in effect since January, and the problems are adding up.

**Leon J. Warshaw:** A problem we are running into regarding women applicants who are already pregnant is the waiting period required by many insurance plans before new employees become eligible for health benefits. In many companies these have been eliminated so that eligibility for benefits starts on the day of employment, but I've heard of a few instances in which their reinstituting is being considered. These would be applicable to all health benefits so that pregnancy is not being treated differently. One way of reinstitution the waiting period is to have a "probationary" period during which new employees are not eligible for benefits of any kind. Of course, this is being resisted by the unions, especially those that have bargained for and won first-day coverage. The point is that this is still a fluid give-and-take situation; this issue is not yet resolved.

**Stillman:** Under the new law, employers can't reduce existing benefits to comply with the pregnancy law until October 31, 1979. Where there is an existing union contract, the freeze lasts until the contract expires. But I too know of at least five employers who do have probationary and conditional clauses in mind—not immediately, but eventually they plan to institute them.

**Marcus B. Bond:** AT&T and many large companies have a form of what we call a leave of absence for anticipated disability. This allows for a period of unpaid leave for the person who is able to work—not disabled—but whom we feel it is not good judgment to require to work. We provide the unpaid leave, and when confinement starts, will begin to pay disability benefits. As for the woman who is eight months pregnant and comes in applying for a job, the letter of the law may say that we cannot refuse to hire her if she's a typist and she knows how to type. But as a matter of practical experience, a number of companies do have some sort of more general rule that requires an expectation of tenure in the job when you hire someone. In our case it's based on the amount of training required for the job. In other words, if we hired a woman who's eight months pregnant for a sales representative position, she would be able to finish only half her training before going into labor, presumably. And that is not considered good business by our business people.

**Louise B. Tyrer:** Assuming that a woman is a successful pole climber and then becomes pregnant, do you have any requirements that she report her pregnancy promptly or concerning how long she may be eligible to continue the activity during her pregnancy?

**Bond:** We handle those cases on an individual basis. Women are supposed to tell their supervisors when they're pregnant. If it is an outside craft job or any other with potential hazards, the supervisor normally requests the Medical Department to make an evaluation. We would look into whether the woman's health is normal and whether the pregnancy is normal, and then make some judgments based on the kind of work she does, correlating it with her health and perhaps at that point talking to the attending obstetrician. In many instances the attending physicians have thought they didn't want the woman to work at all in those jobs after the pregnancy was diagnosed, two or three months along. In other instances, if everything else was favorable, we would let them continue the job as long as they were comfortable doing it—up until, maybe, four or four-and-a-half months when the uterus gets up out of the pelvis and could pose an actual physical hazard.

In regard to the details of placement, we don't think we'll have any trouble. I do not consider it my job or that of our other physicians to try to keep pregnant women from getting benefits for disability. That's not my business. And I treat them the same as I did when I was in private practice, the same way we handle any other employee's medical problem. We will generally agree with and go along with the attending physician, but sometimes we won't, just as we might not agree in the case of a person with a bad knee or back. In cases of disagreement we'll talk directly with the physician and tell him or her what we think, and perhaps also get in a consulting obstetrician if we think that's appropriate. This is exactly how we handle all other such judgments and rarely will there be unique problems, I believe. We will have as our general rule the one that ACOG put out: we wouldn't consider a normal woman with a normal pregnancy routinely disabled prior to the onset of labor. We will reassign women who do physically stressful jobs at some point during their pregnancies; if we cannot reassign them or don't have enough jobs, we'll pay them benefits.

# Non-Medical Issues Presented by the Pregnant Worker*

Leon J. Warshaw, M.D.

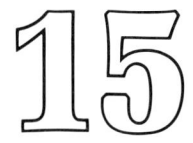

# 15

Several years ago, I was privileged to serve as chairman of a small group of extraordinarily knowledgable and hardworking occupational physicians and obstetricians who were concerned about the health of the pregnant worker and the child she was bearing. We were helped by a dedicated staff provided by the American College of Obstetricians and Gynecologists (ACOG), financial support from the National Institute of Occupational Safety ahd Health (NIOSH), and the generous contributions of two expert panels: one of clinicians and scientists from all of the relevant fields and disciplines; and the other of people who could reflect the views of labor, management, the women's movement, the law and other groups with vested interests in this problem. Quite arbitrarily, we decided to limit our focus to the period of pregnancy and delivery and our concern to the purely clinical aspects of the potential

*Reprinted from *Journal of Occupational Medicine* 21(2), 1978: 403–408, with permission of the publisher.

impact of work and the work environment on the health of the worker and her fetus and the outcome of her pregnancy. For more than a year, we studied and discussed the latest scientific information and the best current practices in obstetrics and occupational medicine and, finally, produced the report, "Guidelines on Pregnancy and Work," that was published by ACOG in 1977 and subsequently reprinted by NIOSH.[1]

Aimed primarily at the physician providing prenatal and obstetrical care, the guidelines offer a format for assembling the necessary information about the health of the pregnant worker and her fetus, the status of her pregnancy and the potential hazards of her job. Then, they provide a logic for using that information to develop the most appropriate recommendations about whether or not she should continue to work and any job changes that might make her work less hazardous and less burdensome. Limited information about specific occupational hazards was included—as expected, some of this is already out-of-date. Nevertheless, the validity of the philosophy and the logic embodied in the guidelines is unimpaired. I commend them to those concerned about any aspect of pregnancy and work.

This presentation will focus on some of the problems and issues that, by design, were not covered in the guidelines. Those who expect definitive solutions will be disappointed; they just do not exist. Scientific information about the influence of environmental exposures on reproductive capacity, child bearing, and the health of the fetus is very limited and much of what we have is based on anecdote and inference whose validity is subject to challenge. The issues are sensitive and fraught with emotion; this leads to dogmatic, doctrinaire attitudes and adversarial positions that make rational discussion difficult, if not impossible. We are in the throes of a social revolution marked by new concepts and changing value judgements with respect to women's rights, the meaning of work and employers' responsibilities to their workers and the consumers of their goods and services. These are reflected in a profusion of laws and regulations that are often confusing and sometimes conflicting.

I have no solutions to offer, but since decisions will not wait, it is my hope that an objective discussion of the problems will facilitate acceptable compromises that will hold until definitive solutions can be evolved.

## The Pregnant Worker

In the words of the guidelines, "a normal woman with a normal pregnancy and a normal fetus in a job presenting no greater potential hazards than those encountered in normal daily life in the community may continue to work without interruption until the onset of labor, and may resume working several weeks after an uncomplicated delivery."

This is applicable to the great majority of women in the work force.

There are, however, some jobs that a pregnant woman cannot perform and there are some that she should not attempt because they involve exposures that are hazardous to her and her fetus or endanger the progress of her pregnancy. There is some work that a well-conditioned pregnant woman who has learned the knack of the job can continue to perform but which should not be attempted by a pregnant woman to whom it would be an entirely new activity. In most instances, the determination that a pregnant woman should not continue in a particular job can be made with reasonable validity only after careful consideration of the stage of her pregnancy, the state of her health, the condition of the fetus, and the kinds and amounts of the hazards to which she would be exposed. An additional consideration is the possibility that these hazards can be eliminated or satisfactorily controlled or that she can be temporarily transferred to another job or location in which they do not occur. If this cannot be done, she might have to stop working.

There are some pregnant women who are quite capable of continuing to work at a particular job without any significant risk. Yet, because of minor discomfort, a desire to stop working or a disinclination to accept reassignment, they seek to have themselves declared "disabled" in order to claim monetary or other benefits. The evaluation of such disability is sometimes quite evident, but most of the time it requires individualized consideration of the particular constellation of circumstances presented by the pregnant worker at the particular time.

Either judgement (that the pregnant woman may work or is disabled) raises a host of non-medical problems. Is the judgement valid or merely an excuse for discrimination? If disabled, what benefits are available to help pay for health care services and to maintain her income? Will her right to return to her job with no loss of seniority or other benefits be maintained? For how long? If temporarily transferred to a job with a lower rate of pay, will she retain her high pay rate and the levels of benefits it provides? Will her transfer be blocked if it involves bumping a co-worker with equal or greater seniority?

Such issues can only be resolved on a case by case basis within the framework of objectivity, fairness, and equity and in accord with established policies, negotiated agreements and relevant laws and regulations.

## Reproductive Capacity

Successful human reproduction requires mature, healthy male and female germ cells, bringing them together through adequate and timely sexual performance, and the proper implantation of the fertilized egg cell. In recent years, we have become painfully aware that environmental exposures may affect these processes and, it is becoming increasingly evident, this can occur in men as well as women.

Sexual activity is strongly influenced by emotional, cultural and physical factors. Marital counselors report that over 50 percent of apparently happily married couples have sexual "hang-ups." Yet, Shakespeare observed that alcohol increases desire but inhibits performance, pharmacologists have noted that certain drugs affect sexual capability, and recent data indicate that impotence may occur in men exposed to toxic agriculture chemicals.

Over 2,000 genetic disorders have been identified. They represent inherited chromosomal abnormalities that can cause fetal wastage, anatomic malformations and developmental disorders. Some are carried by females, some by males, and some by either or both sexes. However, chromosomal damage can also be produced by environmental agents—mutagens—and, presumably, lead to similar effects. At the same time every test system has a spontaneous mutation rate, i.e., a low level background rate of mutation that appears in the absence of known mutagens. Time does not permit a discussion of the implications of chemical mutagenesis; for this, refer to the recent paper by Claxton and Barry.[2]

Human fertility is poorly understood. Diminished fertility and sterility are more easily demonstrated in males but in many instances of infertility, no abnormality can be detected in either partner. Even conception is no guarantee of successful reproduction since over one-third of early embryos fail to survive.[3] While environmental exposures can cause loss of fertility, much more research is needed to delineate the frequency and the magnitude of such effects.

The point here is that exclusion of women from exposure to agents that affect reproductive capacity will not solve this problem. Male workers must be protected as well. The critical problem is that we do not know which chemicals and physical agents affect reproductive capacity or, for those that do, the levels to which exposure must be reduced to obviate such effects. Laboratory studies require extrapolation to man which is not always reliable while the validity of some human studies may be challenged on the basis of sample size and selection, accuracy of exposure records, method of statistical analysis and adequacy of controls. Human monitoring may involve procedures that are unpleasant, somewhat hazardous or culturally unacceptable while epidemiologic studies raise questions of invasion of privacy. Nevertheless, it is desirable to eliminate exposures of both men and women to agents known to have or to be highly suspect of having such effects or, when this is not possible, to monitor exposures to them to maintain the lowest possible level compatible with the circumstances.

## Child-Bearing Capacity

A comprehensive review of current knowledge by Messite and Bond[4] makes it quite clear that normal women are no more susceptible to work related exposures than their male counterparts. However, pregnancy changes this. Hazards that the normal woman might tolerate with impunity threaten the progress of the pregnancy or the development of the fetus. For example, the pregnant woman, her fetus and the newborn infant are particularly vulnerable to the effects of low concentrations of carbon monoxide.[5]

The fetus is most susceptible to toxic exposures during the earliest weeks of pregnancy—the crucial period for organ formation—even before the signs of pregnancy appear or it can be detected by any currently available tests. About 15 percent of recognized pregnancies abort spontaneously, and among those surviving to birth, about 3 percent manifest developmental defects. With increasing age, another 6 percent become detectable.[3] A growing list of environmental agents is being implicated in this "fall-out" and increasingly it is being appreciated that the levels of exposure that lead to such effects may be considerably lower than those regarded as safe for adults.

The ideal solution is to make the workplace safe for all workers, even those who are pregnant, and for the fetus as well, but this is purely theoretical at this time. We don't have the necessary information, we don't have the technical capability, and the cost is often prohibitive.

When possible, the employer should make adjustments in the job to make it safer and less burdensome for the pregnant worker. When these are inadequate or not feasible, she may have to be temporarily transferred to a different job. When none is available, she may have to be placed on maternity leave.

Some employers with women in jobs where potentially toxic exposures are unavoidable require them to report for reassignment at the first indication of pregnancy. Other employers, following the rule suggested by Swartz and Reichling,[6] assume that women in the reproductive years may be pregnant unless it can be proved otherwise and arbitrarily exclude them from certain jobs.

These attempted solutions raise many issues: policies for medical transfer, retention of pay rate if transferred to a lower paying job, seniority rights and "bumping," definition of maternity leave and the eligibility for disability benefits. The exclusion of pregnant workers and women of child-bearing age from jobs for which they would otherwise be qualified raises accusations of discrimination. The mandatory reporting of early pregnancy and requiring proof of inability to bear children have been alleged to be invasions of privacy.

The multiplicity of government agencies involved and the lack of clarity and consistency among their regulations and rulings add to the confusion. The Occupational Safety and Health Administration (OSHA) has regulatory authority to protect workers from occupational hazards but is severely handicapped by the fact that mutagenic and teratogenic information has been recorded for less than 1 percent of the 16,000 chemicals listed in the Registry of Toxic Effects of Chemical Substances, and much of that is not yet validated for humans. Under the Toxic Substances Control Act of 1976, the Environmental Protection Agency is required to ban or restrict the use of any chemical presenting an "unreasonable risk" of injury to health or the environment. A generally acceptable definition of "unreasonable risk" has yet to emerge. The Equal Employment Opportunity Commission is charged to protect the employment rights of women but has yet to set a policy on discriminatory practices related to pregnancy and risks of fetal damage.

Employers are being whipsawed by a "catch 22" situation in which they are subject to complaints and claims no matter what policy they establish. Unions, too, are facing a dilemma. They want to protect the rights of their female members but this might result in their exposure to potentially toxic hazards.

Employers are rightfully concerned about their potential liability for alleged intrauterine injury to the fetus. Awards to adult workers are limited by workers' compensation laws but suit can be brought on behalf of a child. Case law is ambivalent about the legal status of a stillborn fetus within the wrongful death statute but recovery for prenatal injuries suffered any time after conception by a child who was born alive is permitted under Common Law.[7] In a recent malpractice case, the Illinois Supreme Court ruled that a child may have an action for injuries resulting from damage inflicted on its mother years before it was even conceived.[8] The pathetic plight of the Thalidomide babies and reports that, in a country not known for generous legal settlements, the British distributor of that drug paid out over $50 million in awards to the victims of its teratogenic effects, provide ample motivation to protect female employees from such risks.

As mentioned earlier, there are no definitive solutions. Decisions will have to be made on a case by case basis balancing one issue against another. In the absence of validated information, policies, regulations and rules will be promulgated and standards set on the basis of debate and discussion. Union representatives and environmentalists will push for more stringent and rigidly enforced controls. Advocates for women's rights will argue against any limitations of job opportunity and earning capacity. Industry will opt for more lenient standards and voluntary compliance. Hopefully, the result will be responsive to the most reasoned rather than the most strident voices.

I do, however, have some recommendations to offer:

1. The health of the worker and her child and of future generations should always be given prime consideration. In the absence of firm scientific proof, evaluation of risk will necessarily be based on extrapolation, inference and assumption. It should be tilted toward wider rather than narrower margins of safety.
2. Since no standard or rule is likely to protect all people, there should be sufficient flexibility to provide for those at the extremes of the distribution curve.
3. Each worker should have access to the best available advice with respect to family planning and each pregnant worker should have proper prenatal and obstetrical care by health professionals with knowledge of the effects of work exposures on the course of the pregnancy and its outcome. This will be facilitated by providing them with the ACOG Guidelines and having the principles they embody accepted as a standard of practice.
4. A system should be developed to provide workers with understandable, objective and timely information about potential workplace hazards and training in their recognition and control or advoidance. In a recent paper, Blum[9] describes the statutory duty of employers for supplying workers with such information and notes a trend to make failure in this duty an independent cause of legal action, entirely apart from any consideration of injury.
5. An education program should be aimed at all female workers of child-bearing capacity and a special effort made to reach those who are pregnant. It should provide information and motivation to avoid or control the hazards they might encounter in their home life, personal habits and recreational and community activities: e.g., alcohol, cigarette smoking, use of drugs and medications, and exposure to household chemicals.
6. Research should be expanded and accelerated in the toxic effects of known and new chemicals and their dose-response relationships, individually and in combinations. New technology should be developed and put in place for minimizing exposures, monitoring their levels in the workplace and detecting toxic effects in workers as early as possible. The results of this research and their implications should be divulged in appropriate fashion to the workers who may have been exposed and to occupational health professionals.

Reduction of risk and control of potential hazards should outweigh the preservation of trade secrets.

7. Full information should be given to each worker about her own situation and the relative merits of alternative courses of action so that she can participate in any decisions relating to herself and her job. When decisions have to be imposed, their rationale should be explained and honest responses made to any challenges she might offer. Proper written policies should be elaborated and published, preferably with involvement of and endorsement by any unions, as guidelines for such decisions. Both management and labor have been guilty of pursuing vested interests at the expense of the worker, sometimes without her knowledge. Such exploitive behavior should be exposed, decried and corrected.

8. Companies and unions should endorse the codes of professional ethics recently promulgated by the American Occupational Medical Association and the American Association of Occupational Health Nurses and insist that all health professionals employed or retained by them conform to their precepts.

All of this is eminently possible when employers are sophisticated and affluent enough to hire properly qualified health and safety professionals or when workers are represented by unions that set a higher value on the health of an individual member than on "brownie points" for hard bargaining or guarding against justifiable encroachment on prerogatives. This would cover only a portion of the working population, however. The majority work in nonunionized small plants where both knowledge and sophistication in applying it are sadly lacking, and resources are limited. We must find ways to reach and protect them.

Let me close by urging that women workers, pregnant or not, and their male colleagues as well, be treated with honesty, dignity, equity and compassion. This will not solve all of the problems but it will certainly make it much easier to live with them.

## NOTES

1. American College of Obstetricians and Gynecologists: Guidelines on Pregnancy and Work. Chicago: ACOG Publications, 1977.
2. Claxton, L. D. and Barry, P. Z. Chemical mutagenesis: An emerging issue for public health. Am J Public Health 67:1037–1042, 1977.
3. Human Health and the Environment—Some Research Needs. Research Triangle Park, N.C.: National Institute of Environmental Health Sciences DHEW Publication No. (NIH) 77-1277, 1977, 317 ff.

4. Messite, J. and Bond, M.: Consideration for women at work, in Occupational Medicine—Principles and Practical Applications. Vol 2. C. Zenz (Ed.). Year Book Publishers, in press.
5. Longo, L. D.: The biologic effects of carbon monoxide on the pregnant woman, fetus and newborn infant. *Am I Obstet Gynecol.* 129:69–103, 1977.
6. Swartz, H. M. and Reichling, B. A.: Hazards of radiation exposure for pregnant women. *JAMA* 239:1907–1908, 1978.
7. Simon v. Mullin, 380 A.2d 1353 (Conn. Super. Ct., Nov. 2, 1977).
8. Renslow v. Mennonite Hospital, 367 N.E. 2d 1250 (Ill. Sup. Ct., Aug. 8, 1977; rehearing denied Oct. 3, 1977).
9. Blum, J. D.: Revealing the invisible tort: The employer's duty to warn, in *Health Services and Health Hazards: The Employee's Need to Know.* R. H. Egdahl and D. C. Walsh (Eds.), Springer-Verlag, 1978, pp. 173–181.

## Discussion

**Leon J. Warshaw:** A model that we can look at is Sweden, a country that is a little further advanced in such matters than we are. There are, of course, some differences to be taken into consideration: the size of the country, the make-up of the population, the power of the labor movement, and the regressive personal income tax. It is important to note that they call it "parental" insurance, not maternity insurance. There are two kinds: one for the "acquisition of the child," and the other for child care. The former not only covers delivery but offers the leave when a child of any age is adopted. The benefits are available to both fathers and mothers so long as they have been employed six months prior to that time. Together they're eligible for a total of 210 days of paid disability. Twenty-nine days of maternal disability are allowed after the date of delivery; the rest of the 210 days can be divided any way they choose.

The benefits for child care are based upon the number of children a couple has. They get 12 days a year if they have one child, 15 days a year if they have two. This leave is to be used for caring for a sick child, taking the child to the doctor or a preventive health care clinic, or even going to school to discuss with the teacher how the child is doing. In addition, until the child is 8 years old, either parent has the option of reducing the workday by two hours a day. They don't get paid for it, but may work two hours a day less in order to have the time available to take care of that child.

Of course in making comparisons, we also need to consider such factors as the gross national product, the productivity of the labor force, and the birth rate. I haven't heard of any United States corporations giving paid benefits for paternal leave, but I know that a number are considering it.

## A SCANDINAVIAN SOLUTION?

Sweden and Norway are making concerted efforts to stimulate sharing of household and child-raising responsibilities. Unsatisfied with the traditional model of father as provider for the nuclear family and mother as anchor, both Scandinavian nations are encouraging alternative arrangements for child care.

Since 1974, Sweden has been providing "parental insurance" designed to encourage shared child care responsibilities and to ease the economic pressures that make two parental incomes increasingly important. By reimbursing parents for wages lost when caring for a child, the Swedish government hopes to enable one parent to stay home and care for children in certain situations, such as illness, and to cover their loss of income at that time.

Parental insurance benefits are paid in connection with either the birth or adoption of a child and/or the temporary care of a child; they are payable to the parent who refrains from gainful employment for these reasons. The insurance is financed through social insurance premiums paid by employers and the national budget. Limitations are set by the government in regard to the amount to be paid and the length of leaves of absence, generally 6 months. Also, parents receive 3 additional months of paid leave which can be applied to time off or reduced time anytime until the child(ren) reach the age of 8. That families can choose which parent will stay home and how to allocate their leave time (e.g., half day, whole day) enables them to negotiate their most advantageous arrangement, giving them both control over the various responsibilities in their lives and a livelihood without one parent's being compelled to sacrifice either familial or professional involvement.

Similarly, Norway began encouraging "work sharing" in 1971 as a "strategically important, radical (albeit partial) change toward a more basically gratifying and balanced family and occupational life."* The traditional family patterns were seen as contributing to the isolation of mother and child and the occupational absorption and peripheral position of the father in the family. Work sharing was designed to improve family relationships through dual parenting as well as to suggest possible advantages for the employer. Women's work potential could be better used since they would be released from some household responsibilities, eliminating the common occurrence of women working full-time in two spheres—in the office and at home.

The success of both of these models requires that family life and involvement in child raising be respected by employers as a high priority. The governments of both of these nations have taken firm stands to facilitate the acceptance of these priorities. If one attempts to consider the application of these systems to the United States, attention must be paid to essential differences, for example, the size of the country, its gross national product and birthrate, and government expenditures as a percentage of GNP.

*Erik Gronseth, "Work Sharing: A Norwegian Example," in *Working Couples*, ed. R. Rapaport and Robert N. Rapaport with Janice M. Bumstead (New York: Harper and Row, 1978); Eric Morgenthau, "Dads on Duty," *The Wall Street Journal* (January 29, 1979; and "Fact Sheets on Sweden," (Swedish Institute, January 1979).

**Eleanor Tilson:** It's becoming an issue for collective bargaining.

**Jeanne M. Stellman:** Thank goodness we're still living in a country where we do have social movements and laws that do progress with the changes of ideas. Fifteen years ago you couldn't teach in the schools the day you were found pregnant—you were out that day. Now we've come this far. It's a major step forward. About a year ago, I spent a lot of time rereading labor history and testimony, because it's my feeling that women are the driving wedge for improvement in the industrial conditions generally, ever since the first disability laws were passed for them.

**Iver S. Ravin:** The private physician's role raises the point about our tendency to forget the social aspects of this whole problem and treat maternity leave purely as a medical or a women's right issue. What we're really doing is defaulting on the employer's obligation to set the parameters of our benefits and asking the local obstetricians to make the decision for us as to what benefits our patients should get. We're saying it's a disability, then turning to the obstetrician to tell us how disabled they are for how long. Maybe if we can figure a way to decide what benefits we want, and can set some guidelines, we can take the burden off the obstetricians who obviously aren't equipped for it.

**Kenneth C. Edelin:** We would welcome that.

**Tilson:** Isn't it true that physicians have not really met their responsibilities with respect to health care costs in general—not only on this issue but in others.

**Louise B. Tyrer:** But is it the physician's responsibility? I don't think so. To lay it on physicians is the easy way out.

**Tilson:** But you agree that physicians need some education as to what their role should be in this whole picture?

**Tyrer:** Yes, but I think the social issues need be addressed so the physician has appropriate guidelines. At the present time it's just left to the gut reaction of the physician.

**Tilson:** I agree that that must not happen.

**Ravin:** Can physicians become advocates? The problem is that the patient has his physician, the insurer has his physician. The legal counsel uses some other physicians all the time to testify (though they seldom see a patient)—and it doesn't even matter what the physicians say; the lawyers determine it in the long run. We ought to try to set the limits.

**Robert N. Clyne:** At the risk of being branded an eternal pessimist, I do not share any optimism at all about education of physicians in private practice. As an illustration, some six years ago, there was an editorial in the *Journal of the American Medical Association*, subsequently taken up by others, entitled "Never on Wednesday." It pointed out that 90 percent of employees who've been out on disability return to work on a Monday. They may have been well the previous

Tuesday, but they always come back to work on Monday or the first of the month. So a concerted, all-out educational process was undertaken. But physicians resisted, convinced that another few days off would do no harm. It was a total failure, and I'm talking about billions of dollars that are being wasted because of just that one practice. Now we get into something so emotionally charged as a pregnancy, and say to the woman's physician "Thou must do this, thou shalt not do that." But no way is the private doctor going to change his habits whether he's educated or not.

**Edelin:** We've seen a progression here—how to get women into the work force, and once there, how to advance them up the corporate ladder. We've talked about what happens when they conceive, and how we then—"we" meaning society—should protect them and the fetus. One thing that probably is going to have to be the subject for future discussions about social policy is what happens after that. I think we as a society are going to have to confront the very real issue of what's happening to the children when both parents are working or, as is happening so often now, when there is no father living in the home and the mother is obliged to maintain employment outside the home. In these situations we are seeing more and more reliance on day care centers and other third parties to raise our young children. What is this going to mean for future generations, and what kinds of citizens are we going to have in the future? It is of great concern to me, as I am sure it is of great concern to many of us.

# ISSUES FOR THE FUTURE

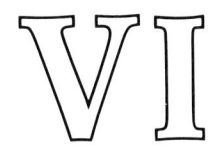

# VI

# Challenges to Corporate Policy

Diana Chapman Walsh

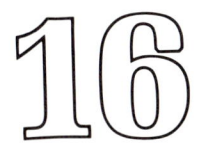

# 16

The subject of this volume has been passed through three successive filters in an effort to distill and clarify the problems it entails. The issues relate specifically to health, to the health of women, and, more particularly, to the health of women employees. These three qualifiers do narrow the field of reference with respect to sheer numbers. Yet the problems remain vexing, partly because the larger issues cannot be entirely separated out.

This final chapter has a dual purpose. First, it reopens broader issues in a brief and merely suggestive way, to serve as a reminder that they need to be reckoned with. Second, it restates the major questions posed in this volume and points to the areas most urgently in need of further attention. The issues are sufficiently intractable that it would be presumptuous to prescribe solutions. To lay the problems out clearly and directly is challenge enough.

Confronted with a complex problem, the best approach, often, is to subject it to reductive analysis—taking it apart and examining separate pieces independently. Then the difficulty comes with the need to reintegrate. But even where this step fails, the reduction process can itself be illuminating.

The special health problems of women workers are undeniably complex. They are part of a social transformation in traditional roles and relationships. They span macroeconomic and manpower policy, medicine, the law, epidemiology, ergonomics, industrial hygiene, biochemistry, and management policy. They fall within the purview of several federal and state statutes and regulatory bodies, which sometimes emit contrary or confusing signals. They bridge gaps between separate functional units within corporations—personnel, finance, and medical, to name just three. Separately and together, the issues animate feminists and abortion activists, as well as the occupational health and labor movements. They demand arbitrary locations along sliding definitional scales (how encompassing is "health," how safe is "safe," how much is "enough"), and bear upon the issues of productivity, mental well-being, family stability, child health and welfare, and the rights and responsibilities of the corporation in society.

For the sake of analysis, this mass of complexity can be arbitrarily reduced to three general categories: (1) a set of issues specific to women who work; (2) a set relating to women's health; and (3) a set pertaining to workers' health. These three categories are neither mutually exclusive nor exhaustive. If one thinks, for example, of a simple matrix with four cells—work/health, men/women—then the three categories include all but the men's work issues. And the four-way matrix begs the issue of interactive effects among work and health, men and women, and also neglects the broader issues that lie beyond work and health per se for society as a whole. But the three categories bear closer scrutiny because of their particular relevance to the special health problems of women workers.

## Issues of Women and Work

*Society does not want women to lead a long life in the home. It is not prepared to support them and cannot give the old style true sanction. Children do not want their parents' lives to be given to them forever. Husbands cannot take the responsibility for wives as an immutable duty, ordained by nature. Women's liberation suits society much more than society itself is prepared to admit. The wife economy is as obsolete as the slave economy.*

ELIZABETH HARDWICK
*Daedalus*[1]

The issues specific to women and work have mostly to do with the failure of public policy to keep pace with the rapidly unfolding social change to which Elizabeth Hardwick refers. Women have problems with the availability of jobs, the quality of available jobs, the flexibility of work, and equality of opportunity in a deteriorating and inhospitable economic climate. The great influx of women into the United States labor force occurred between 1950 and 1976, a time when the economy was able to increase employment by about half.[2] Even so, we have seen in this book the striking occupational segregation which traps women (and minorities) in the poorer quality, lower paying jobs.

Economists are divided on the optimal macroeconomic policy to counter unemployment without worsening inflation and, further, to provide adequate employment for "the overhanging mass of potential job seekers"[3] who go untallied in the labor statistics but would probably search for work if they thought they might find decent jobs. It seems clear that the problem of good jobs and bad jobs is and will remain a pressing issue, especially for women and minorities and, Eli Ginzberg predicts, for social policy as well: "An increasing number of women, because of their heightened attachment to the labor force, will be seeking good jobs and a career, not just any job. . . . The availability of good jobs will become a central issue of public policy."[4]

Also safe is the prediction that the quality of the majority of available jobs will not soon be materially improved by either government action or strategies originating with pressure groups. Approaches arising from within the organization (management and union) are the logical alternative to externally generated change. Thus, the quality of work is likely to remain an issue for corporate personnel policy, and sporadically to reach the corporate agenda in other manifestations or contexts, usually in connection with affirmative action. Again, it may be unrealistic to expect that corporate policy can make numerous jobs intrinsically more satisfying than they now are, although various studies have pointed to specific measures (for example, in the structure of work, or in managerial practices, or group and system design) that corporations could take to improve the quality of work for women and men.[5] Rosabeth Moss Kanter concluded her recent book[6] with a series of concrete recommendations in three broad categories—"opportunity enhancing efforts" (career ladders and review, job redesign and rotation, flexible hours); "empowering strategies" (rewarding superiors for producing successful subordinates, structuring opportunities for women managers to get to know the men who wield power in the firm); and "number balancing strategies" designed to confront the problem of tokenism. But she ends on a less sanguine note:

> Comprehensive approaches are needed . . . yet this conclusion, reached by Harvard Business School researchers as well as radical critics . . . implies widespread system change—virtually the construction of an entirely new system. Such comprehensive change has inherent difficulties and complexities, as well as posing the greatest threat to the greatest number of entrenched power groups and those who like the security of what currently exists . . . the possibilities for reform in large organizations may be inevitably limited.[7]

Inequalities in opportunity, together with conflicts between career objectives and family obligations, are the two most pervasive issues that working women as a group face. Neither is entirely unrelated to health. The strength of that relationship hinges on how far along the causal chain one chooses to search for explanatory variables linked to physical and emotional well-being of working women and their children for generations to come. And both issues complicate the more immediate health concerns. We have seen, for example, how occupational segregation places most women in just those work sites where the government is hardest pressed to enforce its occupational health standards: the small shops scattered throughout light industry with the thinnest profit margins and the least adequate programs of employee benefits and health protection.

## Issues of Women's Health

> *Most controversially, the data may bear out what many critics already claim: namely, that the physicians—who in this study were all male—tend to take illness more seriously in men than in women.*
>
> ARMITAGE, SCHNEIDERMAN AND BASS
> Journal of the American
> Medical Association (JAMA)[8]

How women experience and are treated in medical encounters is one issue of women's health. It is probably connected with another—again a manifestation of job inequality—this time in the health care industry itself. Women currently account for about three-quarters of health workers in the United States, but only about 19 percent of medical school graduates and 15 percent of practicing physicians.[9] This removes them from substantial influence on decisions that shape the health care system. Yet they use the system more than men do, as discussed in chapter 2, for general medical care and the specialized services related to their reproductive function, and often also as custodians of children's health care, or that of older relatives.

Over the past decade a major shift has taken place in childbirth. Psychoprophylactic techniques have gained favor, along with family-centered rather thay physician-orchestrated delivery, greater acceptance of home birth, and so on. This change reflects an increasingly activist consumer role adopted by some women and a new propensity on their part to question the omniscience of the medical profession.[10]

The JAMA study quoted above is a limited and highly tentative look at one of many issues on a neglected research agenda. Solid empirical work could help lay to rest some myths and stereotypes that have conditioned some of the health care that women receive and also could anticipate new issues for the future.[11] For example, widespread attention is only now being paid to the finding that radical mastectomies are a more drastic surgical intervention than necessary for at least some breast cancers. The indications for hysterectomies are being more carefully scrutinized, and there is growing controversy over the possible role of electronic fetal monitoring in increasing the frequency of Caesarian section deliveries. The ramifications for women's and family health of changes in family configurations and in marriage and divorce patterns need attention, as do evolving sexual mores and contraceptive technology, drugs and alcohol dependencies of women, and questions of emotional and sexual development and health. Adequate explanation is lacking for the differences between women and men in health-related behavior and in utilization of health services, and for changes over time in these patterns. The dearth of research on these topics of special concern to women has been attributed to underrepresentation of women in influential positions where research priorities are set.[12]

These empirical questions spill over into the realm of occupational health where, as we have seen, systematic research is badly needed as a basis for corporate and social policy. Whether the object be to validate job-placement tests, as in the AT&T case, to quantify the major risk factors for physical and emotional stress on the job, to compare the impact on children of various day care alternatives, to identify threats to successful reproductive outcomes, or to assess the effect of work on women's longevity (and the reverse), the research task looms large for investigators, whether basic or behavioral scientists.

Health issues can be used politically, socially, or scientifically. The basic question—in the workplace and beyond—is how and where are health issues being used for and against women. When is *protection* merely a code word for withholding opportunity, and when is it a genuine need? Without more information, these remain open questions.

## Issues of Workers' Health

> There is no point in getting into a panic about the risks of life until you have compared the risks which worry you with those that don't—but perhaps should. . . . What we need, therefore, is a list or index of risks and some guidance as to when to flap and when not.
>
> BARON NATHANIEL MAYER VICTOR ROTHSCHILD<br>Wall Street Journal[13]

> Mutagens and carcinogens must be treated with respect; priorities must be set, alternatives examined, and human exposure minimized. We have seen, and will continue to see, the folly of using humans as guinea pigs.
>
> BRUCE N. AMES<br>Science[14]

Questions of scientific priorities in the assessment of risks are the most fundamental unresolved issues in occupational health, coupled, in the absence of scientific certainty, with the employee's need to know. This has been an emphasis of the federal occupational health establishment, which has incorporated into its standards the employer's obligation to maintain and assure employees' access to records of occupational accidents and illnesses that have occurred and of exposure levels to dangerous substances in their workplaces. Results of job-related medical examinations must also be available, subject to the written consent of the worker whose record it is. The fourth volume in the Industry and Health Care series observed that communication serves as a kind of preventive medicine and is, in the case of clear and present danger, widely recognized by industry as a crucial early step to take. As hazards become less immediate and not so easily discerned, consensus breaks down over how much latitude employees actually have in deciding what hazards they will endure on the job and how rationally they will weigh low-probability, long-range risks to their health. There is nearly unanimous agreement, though, on the basic approach advocated by Lord Rothschild and Bruce Ames: the need to develop a sophisticated understanding of the risks to which we are daily subjected—"risk accounting" is Lord Rothschild's notion—so that individuals can go about the business of deciding for themselves "when to flap" and so scientists can establish research priorities that do indeed avoid "the folly of using humans as guinea pigs."

Issues of workers' health are the province of occupational medicine, a profession in some ferment, as described in earlier volumes of the Industry and Health Care series. As the specialty evolved in this country, the organized medical profession carved a sharp line of demarcation between occupational and nonoccupational health care. Industrial medicine was neglected in medical school curricula and residency programs and was isolated in a rather remote professional niche, focusing narrowly on environmental hazards, toxicology, and routine treatment of job-associated illness, injury, and disability. Nonoccupational problems were traditionally off bounds.

That situation is changing and the niche is no longer so remote. The "flowering of the chemical age"[15] since the mid-1950s has given the toxicological and environmental functions greater intrinsic importance, with external impetus from the 1970 Occupational Safety and Health Act (OSHA) and the 1976 Toxic Substances Control Act (TSCA). The greater proportion of slowly developing chronic diseases further undermines the always elusive notion that an illness can definitively be labeled "occupationally induced" or not. The likelihood of some form of national health insurance plan and the steady growth of employer-financed private health insurance reduce the relevance of a disability's origin from the standpoint of whether the employer will pay for associated medical services. The problem of rising health care costs has impelled many corporations to summon all the expertise they can muster, often including the corporate medical director, on an internal cost containment task force. Finally, the newly awakened interest in health promotion and disease prevention—both generally[16] and in the workplace[17]—melds the public health perspective that is part of occupational medicine with the primary care functions that used to lie in the exclusive realm of the private practitioner.

Against this historical backdrop, corporations are sorting out relationships with practicing physicians involved in the certification of disability for pregnancy under the new maternity law. Even if corporations "merely" wanted physicians to reorient their thinking to "ration" disability slips, they would face a delicate persuasive task. But they actually need physicians not policing but functioning in a much more elaborate role, helping to obviate serious potential risks to employees and employers when fertile or pregnant women are exposed to certain kinds of toxic substances in the workplace.

Redefining these relationships—including those with women employees—will take place in highly charged force fields: between women and obstetricians (where there is often a strong bond of loyalty but occasional discord over issues of physician dominance and patronizing or insensitive treatment); between workers and occupational physicians (where there remains a residuum of suspicion over confidentiality, access to information, social control, and paternalistic attitudes); as well as between the law and medicine on the one hand and the law and occupational health on the other.

## The Special Health Problems of Women Workers

When we attempt the reintegration now of the problems specific to the health of women workers, it becomes virtually impossible to get a clean cut, independent of ancillary issues and free of biases or fundamental discord among different visions for the future of work, men, women, and families. From some perspectives, it may be acceptable to consider trading off some safety, some productive efficiency, or some of the firm's profit in the interest of equal opportunity or to sacrifice access to certain kinds of jobs in order to assure safety. From others, these compromises are unthinkable. The indivisibility of the issues makes it exceedingly difficult to move from global objectives on which everyone can agree—healthy children, families, and workers—to practical questions of how to establish and implement policy, allocate resources, choose among conflicting priorities, and assess risks in pursuit of these ends.

For now the best we can do is to identify the major issues remaining to be resolved over the next decade or so in the four health-related areas covered in this book, and to extract a few underlying themes.

### Physical Conditioning and Testing

When corporations such as AT&T embark on a program to move women into nontraditional and physically demanding jobs, they encounter new questions concerning the scope of their responsibilities in the face of competing claims:

- To women employees, how much remedial training should the company offer at what extra expense? How carefully must the firm validate the legitimacy of tests used to screen applicants for the special training? What are the relative merits of training women in the skills needed to perform physically stressful tasks, retooling the tasks to make them easier, or redesigning the jobs to make the physically demanding tasks less essential? What if injury rates increase? Or, if after extensive training the workers decide they liked their old jobs better?

- To male coworkers, how much reverse discrimination can be justified in the hope of righting old wrongs? Under what circumstances is it true that changes for women's sake improve working conditions for all?

- To the public, the taxpayer, the consumer, the stockholder and other investors, is there an obligation to consider, and perhaps try to track, the costs of specific remedial efforts and who ultimately bears them at what levels?

An important feature of the AT&T consent decree was that it imposed on the Bell companies a detailed internal reporting system to monitor their progress toward equal opportunity. The requirement constitutes an unprecedented intrusion by the government into the internal data collection and monitoring system of a corporation.[18] Whether it is a bellwether or merely a symbolic gesture remains to be seen, but it does lend some credence to the notion that social issues—such as women's jobs—will persist during the coming decade as a major testing ground of the division of power between business and government.[19]

As an instrument of power, information—the collection and use of data—will certainly remain a central issue here as it is in all of industry's involvements in health. From industry's role as a payer for employee health benefits there is mounting pressure on the insurance carriers to provide more and better data on how the money is spent (the subject of an earlier volume in the Industry and Health Care series). As "consumers" of health services with a role to play in shaping public policy, planning community facilities, and guiding hospitals through troubled times, some companies, either alone or with neighboring firms, are beginning to look more closely at their employees' experiences and to bring those data to bear on decision making. And especially in industry's provider role, demands for corporate health data are escalating as a consequence of external pressures (from OSHA and TSCA) and internal pressures (for cost-benefit accounting and evaluations of innovative programs like the employee assistance programs treated in another volume of the Industry and Health Care series).

## Emotional Conditioning, Social and Health Needs

Child care and the organization of work are the two principal issues women workers will present to corporations for social and emotional needs. Some women will elect to sacrifice or forgo family in the pursuit of career or career in the name of family; others will look for compromises that allow them to juggle the two roles. The increased proportion of women in the labor force will call attention—in the breach—to the essential social (and economic) roles they have hitherto played in families and communities. As more women earnestly pursue careers, the disruption this may mean for the lives of husbands, fathers, and children could place an appreciable burden on corporations to establish their own programs to fill in the gaps in child care and related social services, or to offer more flexible work arrangements and parental leave policies for women *and* men workers.

## Hazards to Fertility and Reproductive Outcomes

Information, again, is the central issue here. If workers desire autonomy to make decisions concerning occupational exposures, they still depend on the accessibility, reliability, and clarity of the information their employers provide. This, too, is a testing ground between business and government, where the control of data frequently surfaces as a symbol as well as a practical impasse.

On the especially touchy problem of whether or when fertile women should be excluded from hazardous jobs, more research is needed to establish risks for both women and men. As stopgap measures, though, some exclusionary policies are probably unavoidable. The acrimony such policies have engendered in the past suggests that more attention should be paid to the process through which the decision is reached, since women's interests are so inadequately represented in the decision-making hierarchy of both management and labor unions. Part of the decision process involves addressing the question of how to offer appealing and equitable alternatives to the jobs from which certain classes of employees are being excluded.

A longer range research and educational effort will be required to establish the foundations for an index of the risks encountered in daily living and to develop the mechanisms and collective mind-set for systematically "coming to grips with risk." One controversial suggestion is to make it a policy to place older people in the more toxic workplaces, on the theory that these exposures are less likely than with younger people to catch up with them before something else does. Logically the converse of the policy to exclude fertile women from certain jobs, this is a discomforting notion which, nevertheless, probably ought to be discussed openly.

## Pregnancy and Maternity Leave

The immediate issue here is how to implement a sweeping new law, which, like most political products, has its strong and weak points. Opponents fear it has gone too far; proponents regret its failure to meet expectations. Certainly it is causing administrative headaches. How costly it will be for corporations to implement and what, if any, fraction of those costs will be attributable to abuses by women or physicians remains for now an open question, as does the effect it will have on the corporation's relations with women's personal physicians.

## Underlying Themes

Of several generic themes that cut across these four specific topics, the one that stands out is the broad question of information and decision making. Information is crucial as the basis for sound decisions but is also a frequent source of strife. More information needs to be collected, as well as communicated effectively both across subunits of corporations and among corporations, government, and special interest groups. A specific data element that is lacking but that is assumed to be important is the cost of the accommodations being demanded of industry. Actual and potential costs over the short and longer range are often mentioned as a problem, though rarely in specific, quantitative terms. Who actually bears these costs and what the tradeoffs really are is far from clear. This influences the way decisions are reached and who has access to that decision process—perhaps the bedrock issue, and part of a more philosophical question as to the role of corporations in a democratic society and the appropriate balance between public and private controls on corporate activities.

It is easy but not very helpful to simply assert that working women ought to have a greater say in the decisions that affect their lives. One needs to understand the structural problems (where women are in the work force) that mute effective participation and also to consider the mechanisms through which structural changes may occur. Legal mechanisms have been prominent in this discussion—some (such as the AT&T consent decree and the Pregnancy Disability Act) are political or social expressions; others (such as OSHA and TSCA) rest more on scientific foundations. There is the possibility that these are working at cross purposes; individually, they are limited instruments of social policy based on imperfect information and tenuous consensus. For the future, corporations can anticipate a continuation and probably an intensification of current patterns, with pressures building from below as more women enter the work force, erupting occasionally in legal attempts to speed the natural evolutionary process toward greater equality when the perception develops that progress is too slow.

In spite of their complexity, the health problems of women workers are probably more amenable to solution than are the broader social issues they touch. There is at least some basis for hope that acceptable solutions can be gradually evolved in this sphere, possibly with wider applications, for example, by accelerating the rapprochement already occurring between occupational and general medicine, improving the process by which risks of toxic exposures in the workplace are assessed and handled, or calling attention to specific aspects of work that especially stress employees and their families. Certainly the better solutions will be those that improve the working lives of women *and* men. Perhaps the solutions developed in this narrow but challenging sphere can make a contribution to the definition and conceptual underpinnings of corporate social responsibility in the difficult years that lie ahead.

## NOTES

1. Elizabeth Hardwick, "Domestic Matters," *Daedalus* 107 (*A New America?*, Winter 1978): 1, 11.
2. Eli Ginzberg, "The Job Problem," *Scientific American* 237 (November 1977): 45.
3. Ibid., p. 47.
4. Ibid., p. 49.
5. See, e.g., J. Richard Hackman and J. Lloyd Suttle, *Improving Life at Work* (Santa Monica: Goodyear Publishing, 1977).
6. Rosabeth Moss Kanter, *Men and Women of the Corporation* (New York: Basic Books, 1977).
7. Ibid., p. 285.
8. Karen J. Armitage, Lawrence J. Schneiderman, and Robert A. Bass," Response of Physicians to Medical Complaints of Men and Women," *Journal of the American Medical Association* 241 (May 18, 1979): 2186–2187.
9. Barbara Mercado, "Women Have Stake in NH Plan," *The Nation's Health* (August 1979): 8.
10. Boston Women's Health Book Collective, *Our Bodies, Ourselves* (New York: Simon and Schuster, 1971).
11. Virginia Olesen, ed., *Women and Their Health: Research Implications for a New Era*, U.S. Department of Health, Education, and Welfare, Pub. no. (HRA) 77-3138, 1977.
12. Rose Laub Coser, "Why Bother? Is Research On Issues of Women's Health Worthwhile?" in ibid., pp. 3–9.
13. Baron Nathaniel Mayer Victor Rothschild, "Coming to Grips with Risk," *Wall Street Journal* (March 13, 1979): 22.
14. Bruce N. Ames, "Identifying Environmental Chemicals Causing Mutations and Cancer," *Science* 204 (May 11, 1979): 592.
15. Ibid., p. 588.
16. U.S. Surgeon General, *Healthy Americans* (Washington, D.C.: Department of Health, Education, and Welfare, 1979).
17. Office of Health Information and Health Promotion, *Proceedings of the National Conference on Health Promotion Programs in Occupational Settings* (Washington, D.C.: U.S. Department of Health, Education, and Welfare, 1979).
18. Christopher D. Stone, *Where the Law Ends* (New York: Harper and Row, 1975): 203.
19. Nancy Needham Wardell, "The Corporation," *Daedalus* 107 (*A New America?*, Winter 1978): 97–100.

# Appendix

## Conference Participants
"The Special Problems of Women Workers," sponsored by Boston University Health Policy Institute, Boston: June 11–12, 1979

John L. Bauer, Jr., Supervisor, Insurance Benefits, Armco Corporation, Middletown, Ohio

Edward J. Bernacki, M.D., Corporate Medical Director, United Technologies Corporation, Hartford, Connecticut

William J. Bicknell, M.D., Director, Special Health Programs, Boston University, and Medical Director, United Mine Workers of America Health and Retirement Funds, Boston, Massachusetts, and Washington, D.C.

John D. Blum, J. D., Consultant, Harbridge House, Boston, Massachusetts

Leslie I. Boden, Ph.D., Assistant Professor, Harvard School of Public Health, Boston, Massachusetts

Marcus B. Bond, M.D., Corporate Medical Director, American Telephone and Telegraph Company, Basking Ridge, New Jersey

Robert M. Clyne, M.D., Corporate Medical Director, American Cyanamid Company, Wayne, New Jersey

## Appendix

Robert E. Cooke, M.D., President, Medical College of Pennsylvania, Philadelphia, Pennsylvania

Gail E. Costa, Occupational Health Study Director, Rhode Island Group Health Association, Providence, Rhode Island

Stanley P. deLisser, President, The Executive Health Examiners Group, New York, New York

Jean P. Dietz, Staff Reporter, *Boston Globe*, Boston, Massachusetts

Ernest M. Dixon, M.D., Corporate Medical Director, Celanese Corporation, New York, New York

Jean F. Duff, Vice President, General Health Corporation, Washington, D.C.

Kenneth C. Edelin, M.D., Chairman, Department of Obstetrics and Gynecology, Boston University Medical Center, Boston, Massachusetts

Richard H. Egdahl, M.D., Director, Boston University, Center for Industry and Health Care, Boston, Massachusetts

Jean G. French, Dr. P.H., Health Scientist, National Institute for Occupational Safety and Health, Rockville, Maryland

Donald R. Giller, Administrative Director, Occupational Health Service Center, University Hospital, Boston, Massachusetts

William E. R. Greer, M.D., Corporate Medical Director, Gillette Company, Boston, Massachusetts

Marcie G. Grymes, Senior Staff Assistant, General Motors Corporation, Detroit, Michigan

Joyce Hogan, Ph.D., Research Scientist, Advanced Research Resources Organization, Washington, D.C.

Edwin T. Holmes, J.D., Counsel, Health Insurance Association of America, New York, New York

Susan C. Karp, Benefits Specialist, Citibank, New York, New York

Bruce W. Karrh, M.D., Corporate Medical Director, E.I. DuPont de Nemours, Wilmington, Delaware

Frank J. Kefferstan, II, M.D., Corporate Medical Director, John Hancock Mutual Life Insurance Company, Boston, Massachusetts

Ann Lebowitz, Writer/Research Associate, Boston University, Center for Industry and Health Care, Boston, Massachusetts

Pamela A. Koo, Manager, Special Projects and Member Services, Washington Business Group on Health, Washington, D.C.

Donna Morrison, R.N., Vice President, Executive Health Examiners, National Health Services, Inc., Washington, D.C.

Warrie Price, Trustee, Boston University Medical Center, Boston, Massachusetts

Iver S. Ravin, M.D., Medical Director, Boston Edison, Boston, Massachusetts

## Appendix

Richard R. Reilly, Ph.D., Project Manager, American Telephone and Telegraph Company, Basking Ridge, New Jersey

Anthony W. Rogers, J.D., Director of Legal Studies, Boston University, Center for Industry and Health Care, Boston, Massachusetts

Jeanne M. Stellman, Ph.D., Executive Director and Division Chief, Women's Occupational Health Resource Center, New York, New York

Nina G. Stillman, J.D., Attorney, Vedder, Price, Kaufman and Kammholz, Chicago, Illinois

Deborah A. Stone, Ph.D., Assistant Professor, Political Science, Massachusetts Institute of Technology, Cambridge, Massachusetts

Eleanor Tilson, Vice President and Administrator, United Storeworkers Union, New York, New York

Louise B. Tyrer, M.D., Vice President for Medical Affairs, Planned Parenthood Federation of America, New York, New York

Stephen J. Varholy, Associate Director, Human Resources Division, United States General Accounting Office, Washington, D.C.

Patricia A. Walker, Director, Medical Records, Tabershaw Occupational Medicine Association, Rockville, Maryland

Christopher Walsh, Ph.D., Professor, Chemistry and Biology, Massachusetts Institute of Technology, Cambridge, Massachusetts

Diana Chapman Walsh, Director, Industry Health Program Evaluation, Boston University, Center for Industry and Health Care, Boston, Massachusetts

Leon J. Warshaw, M.D., Vice President and Corporate Medical Director, Equitable Life Assurance Society of the United States, New York, New York, on loan to the Office of the Mayor, City of New York

Glen Wegner, M.D., J.D., Medical Director, Boise Cascade Corporation, Boise, Idaho

Stephen M. Weiner, J.D., Director, Boston University Center for Law and Health Sciences, Boston, Massachusetts

3 1222 00107 9345

DATE DUE

MAR 24 1982

JAN 07 1989

OCT 12 1995

GAYLORD                                      PRINTED IN U.S.A.

NO LONGER THE PROPERTY
OF THE
UNIVERSITY OF R.I. LIBRARY